HOPE AND LIGHT IN THE DARKNESS

A STORY BY THE COUNTRY DOCTOR

CARL MATLOCK MD

MATLOCK PUBLISHING

Hope and Light in the Darkness: A Story by the Country Doctor

Copyright 2020 by Carl Matlock

Published in the United States by Matlock Publishing, Mitchell, Indiana

ISBN: 978-0-9600521-8-9 Paperback

ISBN: 978-0-9600521-7-2 eBook

Cover and Interior Design by Carl Matlock

Editing by Christy Distler, Avodah, Editorial Services

Images by Shutterstock.com, Used by Permission

First Edition

❋ Created with Vellum

This Book is dedicated to the memory of my parents, Carl Joseph and Christina Maxine (Evans) Matlock. They first taught me about faith and hope by pointing me to 'The Light' in the writings of the Holy Bible.
Thanks once more to my wonderful first editor, Janet Sue (Speer) Matlock, my loving wife of fifty years. She faithfully reads and critiques my initial endeavors. Sometimes, my first works never see the light of day after she offers valuable insights for my consideration.

ACKNOWLEDGMENTS

I wish to express my gratitude to Christy Distler and Avodah Editorial Services for improving my final manuscript for publication. Her contribution greatly added to the quality of the finished work, *Hope and Light in the Darkness, A Story by the Country Doctor.*

PREFACE

Hope and Light in the Darkness, A Story by the Country Doctor, is my fourth work of medical fiction. The only actual names given are those of my family members. They lived these stories with me. I have taken care to hide the identity of other people named in my books.

Please note that the treatments of the past are not recommendations for similar medical conditions today. Medicine has changed drastically as computers replaced paper charts and technology advanced at a dizzying pace in diagnostic and treatment innovations, both medical and surgical. The primary care specialties continue to be challenging for this very reason.

I based the accounts in this book on my interactions with thousands of patients encountered in forty-seven years of medical practice. I attained board certification in both Family Medicine and Emergency Medicine, thus giving me a wide range of experience. The characters and situations in my stories make up a composite of many patients and events. I genuinely loved living the life of a medical doctor, retiring in 2018 due to health issues.

If this work gives the reader a flavor of the practice of rural medicine nearly fifty years ago, I will have succeeded in one of my goals, that of writing about a simpler and friendlier time of life.

I'm thankful for the opportunity I had of practicing medicine in rural Indiana. I cherish the memories from those days. Please join me in hospital rounds, house calls, office visits, and delivering babies. It was a world that will never exist again. Come with me and see!

Hope and Light in the Darkness

A Story by the Country Doctor

Carl Matlock, MD

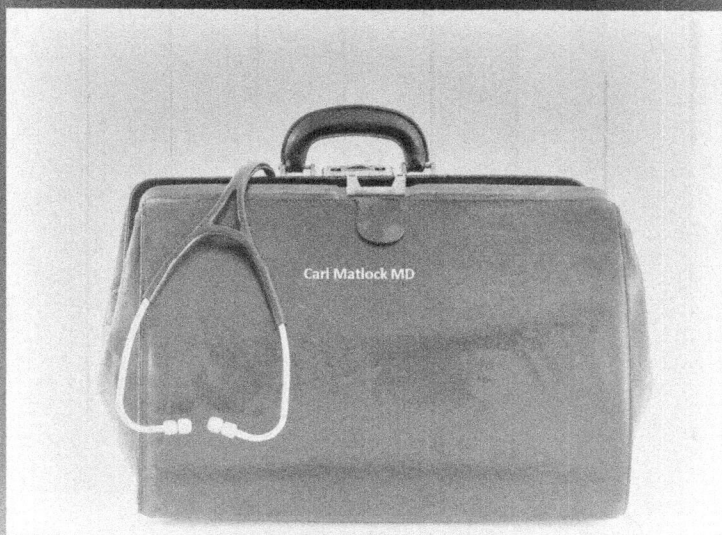

Carl Matlock MD

CHAPTER 1—GASTRIC TUMOR

"What's the verdict, Doc? Do you think I'll live a while?"

I gazed at Jack O'Conner seated across from me in my office in Glen Oaks, Indiana, hesitating as I grasped for the right words. It's never easy to inform a patient and friend of an ominous laboratory finding. He had been one of my first patients when I began practice four years ago in the summer of 1973. Friendly and outgoing, he often stopped to chat while walking his regular mail delivery route in town. My mind wandered back to two weeks ago when Jack came in for an acute visit.

Noticing my reticence, Jack continued his attempt at lighthearted banter. "What about it? An old goat like me can't be seriously ill." He paused and furrowed his brow. "Can I?"

"I'm sorry. I don't mean to put you off, but the upper GI you had done revealed a problem."

Leaning forward in his chair, Jack swallowed hard and then cleared his throat. "What kind of problem? I'm sick a lot, but I'm not having much pain."

"There is a tumor causing partial obstruction of your distal stomach, the part near the outlet into the intestines."

Jack gazed at the floor and squeezed his hands together until the knuckles whitened. "I was afraid of something like this. Cancer runs in my family. Why should I be an exception?"

"Wait a minute. Don't reach a conclusion until we have more information. I don't have a diagnosis yet. There is a tumor, possibly malignant, and it's a surgical problem. Your stomach isn't obstructed, but if the tumor grows a little more, it soon will be. Whether it's cancer or a benign growth, I can't say. The x-ray reveals a blockage large enough to slow the emptying of partially digested food from the stomach, resulting in nausea and intermittent vomiting."

He looked up at me. "You're trying to tell me I need to see a surgeon soon, aren't you?"

"Yes. Sorry to seem so hazy in my explanation. It's never easy to tell a friend he needs to see a surgeon."

"It's okay, Doc. We're still friends. The reason my family and I come to you is that you never attempt to hide the truth from us. Believe me, we appreciate that about you." The color had drained from his face, and he took out a handkerchief and mopped sweat from his brow. "Well, what's the next step?"

Alarmed, I leaned forward and placed my hand on his knee. "Are you getting sick again?"

"Yeah. I think I may vomit."

I opened the door and called down the hallway, "Donna, I need your help." Then I assisted Jack onto the examination table so he could lie down.

Within seconds, Donna bustled into the room, took in the situation with a glance, and grabbed an emesis basin from beneath the sink.

Jack turned onto his right side and began dry heaving.

Donna moistened a washcloth and sponged his forehead, wiping away rivulets of sweat and whispering words of comfort as he vomited a slight amount of clear fluid into the basin I held for him.

Donna glanced at me. "Tigan?"

"Sure. Draw up 200 mg stat."

Jack shivered a little. "What's Tigan?"

"It's an injection to relieve your nausea. It makes some people drowsy. Is your family in the waiting room?"

"No. I came alone today, but my wife is home. I didn't want Janie to come in case the news wasn't good. Guess I made a mistake, huh?"

I nodded. "Guess you did. She has to be involved in your care. Don't hide it from her or your family. They need to know."

Jack grimaced as he rolled onto his back. "You're right. She already suspects the worst. I heard her talking to one of her friends on the phone last week, sharing her suspicions."

Donna returned with the injection. "Jack, I'll need you to pull down your pants. This goes in the hip. There's more muscle there."

"Okay. Okay. Don't rush me." He turned again, muttering about a certain sadistic nurse.

Donna hunched her shoulders and glared at him. "I can go get a bigger, blunt needle."

Jack winked at me as he regained his sense of humor. "Just kidding. I wouldn't want anyone else to give me the shot, especially not Doc. He wouldn't be as gentle."

Donna jammed the needle into his hip and depressed the plunger after first aspirating to be sure she had not hit a blood vessel. Jack tugged his pants up and rolled onto his back once more, giving a wan smile to Donna.

She grinned. "That's more like it. A nurse wants to feel appreciated."

"Could you stay with Jack for a few minutes?" I said to her. "I'll have Christine call Janie to come get him. Then I'll see the patients you already have in other rooms while we wait for her."

Donna winked. "I'll be glad to remain here and make sure there are no more derogatory remarks about nurses."

Jack managed another weak grin, then gave her hand a quick squeeze. "Who will keep you on your toes if I don't?"

I left them trading friendly insults and went to tell Christine to call Janie O'Conner to the office, then continued seeing the last patients of the day. It was the closing hour, and I wanted to have plenty of time to speak with Jack and Janie after everyone else departed for home. Christine had left the front desk to assist me while Donna stayed with Jack, and we soon finished.

It was almost 5:30 p.m. when Janie rushed in the front door, out of breath and with her face flushed. Their eighteen-year-old son, William, followed her, shaking his head. He looked perplexed and worried.

Christine rushed to the waiting room to meet them.

"Hi, Christine," Janie said. "I'm sorry to take so long. William's old jalopy wouldn't start. I had to call him home from basketball practice at school to help me."

He sighed. "Mom, you flooded the carburetor. You left the choke out and pumped the accelerator too many times. And it's a '49 Chevy, not just an old jalopy."

Janie shook her head. "Whatever. I still don't know what you see in that old black, scarred, beat-up excuse for a car."

"Wheels, Mom. Wheels!"

Observing that both were overly excited, Christine intervened. "It's okay. We're glad you got here safe and sound. Now if you'll follow me, we'll go see your hubby. He's with Doc and feeling better after a shot for nausea. Donna took him into exam room 4, which doubles as Doc's office and conference room. The chairs are much more comfortable, and Mr. O'Conner is feeling better, sitting up in a soft brown leather chair and sipping lemon-lime Gatorade from our refrigerator." Exercising her usual loquacious gift of banter, Christine regaled them with non-stop entertainment all the way down the hall and into exam room 4.

As she opened the door, she was still talking. "As I was saying ..." Her voice trailed off at seeing that Jack and I were listening to the conversation. Christine turned about into the hallway and finished, "Never mind. Tell you later. I need to help Donna clean the rooms before we go home."

Jack shook his head, smiling. "That girl is a talking tornado and non-stop chatterbox, but I wouldn't change her for the world."

Janie gave a nervous laugh as she took a seat while William preferred

4

to stand statue-like beside his mother. She heaved a worried sigh, then asked, "What's wrong with my husband, Doc? Is it serious?"

Jack nodded for me to inform his family.

"He has a partial obstruction near the outlet of the stomach. It's an abnormal growth or tumor, but we don't have a diagnosis yet as to type of tissue."

Janie blinked back tears. "It's cancer, isn't it?"

William patted his mother on the shoulder.

"It may be, but we won't know until a surgeon does more testing."

Jack stared at the floor as I handed a box of tissues to Janie, whose tears slid down her face. He cleared his throat and looked up. "Janie, stop making a fuss. This is another hurdle in life we'll get through together. I'll be okay."

She shook her head. "You don't know that, Jack O'Conner. I don't want to lose you."

"Folks, one thing at a time. Any surgery is potentially serious, but let's talk about a plan to tackle the problem." That got their attention, and they quieted and looked at me in anticipation. "First, Jack needs to see a surgeon for a definitive diagnosis."

"How about Dr. Hendrick? You sent me to him two years ago for a hernia repair, and I like him."

"That's just who I had in mind. He does endoscopy and open abdominal surgery. He can do endoscopy and biopsy the tumor. Then we'll know how to best approach the problem. Agreed?"

Janie dried her tears and blew her nose. "Agreed. The sooner the better."

Jack nodded. "I trust you and Dr. Hendrick. That will be fine with us." He looked at his family. "We need to call Lynn tonight and let her know, or she won't forgive us. But I'll be the one to tell her. Understood?"

William nodded.

"Of course, dear," Janie said. "Whatever you say." She looked back at me. "Lynn finished her second year at IU and is taking a summer course on the Bloomington campus. She's still a daddy's girl."

Jack beamed with pride. "Doing good in her pre-med studies too, Doc. I'm real proud of her."

"You have every right to be proud," I said. "She's a fine young lady and will make a skilled physician. Now, before you go, do you have any more nausea?"

"No. That shot helped a lot."

"In that case, I'll write you a prescription for Tigan capsules 250 mg, and Tigan suppositories 200 mg just in case you can't keep the capsules down. As you said, you aren't eating much. For now, stick with soups, Gatorade, tea, and broth until I can get you in to see Dr. Hendrick. I'll personally call his office and see if he'll work you into the schedule tomorrow because of your symptoms and the UGI findings."

William moved to his father's side to offer support as Jack stood up, still a little shaky.

Jack smiled at me once more as he left with his family. "Thanks to you and your staff, I feel better than I have in the last twenty-four hours. Tell Donna and Christine thanks for me. I appreciate all your help."

The girls had already left, and I stood on the porch stoop waving as Jack and Janie drove off in their 1974 Chevy Caprice. William warmed up his jalopy, pulled onto the street emitting a dense, choking cloud of exhaust from his tail pipe, and then roared off behind them, his engine backfiring like a double-barreled shotgun.

Watching them head home, I shook my head. I didn't have a reassuring feeling about Jack's diagnosis or his prognosis.

CHAPTER 2—DIAGNOSIS AND PROGNOSIS

The next day, Jack and Janie sat in an examination room in Glen Falls awaiting consultation. Jack drummed on Rob Hendrick's desk beside his chair, beating out a syncopated rhythm with his fingers. Janie fidgeted in the chair beside him, then snapped, "Stop making that annoying racket. You're getting on my nerves."

"Sorry. I didn't know I was even doing it. Guess I'm tense. And you seem to be flipping through that fashion magazine while you stare at the wall. I haven't seen you look at one page for a couple of minutes."

Janie closed the copy of *Vogue*. "You're right. I'm doing the same thing you are, Jack, trying to relieve pressure before I explode. If Dr. Hendrick doesn't get here soon, I believe I'll scream. We had to wait until this afternoon to see him, and now he's tied up in another operation. I think he should keep the appointments he has before starting another surgery."

"Now, dear, be reasonable. His receptionist said he was doing an emergency appendectomy. What if our son needed an emergency operation?"

Janie threw her copy of *Vogue* back on the magazine table. "I know.

I'm not being fair, but I don't want to lose you. I need to know what happens next."

Just then, the exam door opened. "I'm so sorry, Jack," Rob Hendrick said. "Didn't mean to keep you waiting, but a little boy had a ruptured appendix when he got to the emergency room."

Jack nodded. "That's okay, Doctor. I'm glad you worked me in today."

"And I'm glad you waited. Most of the patients rescheduled for later in the week, but I wanted to see you today."

"Sure, I realize it may not be good news, but shoot the works."

Rob pulled up a chair across from them. "I've reviewed the UGI done last week, and I really can't tell the diagnosis yet, but as you know, you have a tumor and it could be cancer. I won't hide anything from you."

Jack nodded as Janie sat, body rigid, hands clasped together tightly. He held out his left hand until she noticed and accepted his hand with a gentle squeeze.

Dr. Hendrick looked from one to the other. "This is never easy, folks, but I want you to be very clear on the next steps to take."

"It's okay. I want it straight from you," Jack said. "I've a family to consider. Maybe you remember William and Lynn. They're eighteen and twenty now."

"I haven't met William, but Lynn came to my office to observe my practice before she started her college studies. She's a fine girl. Dr. Matlock told me later that she spent time in his office too and decided on a medical career. She'll make a fine physician. If I can ever help her, tell her to contact me. I'm always glad to help young people get an excellent start in the medical field."

Janie smiled for the first time. "Thanks. That means a lot to us."

Jack winked at Dr. Hendrick and gave Janie's hand another squeeze.

"First, I want to emphasize that the etiology or exact tissue diagnosis cannot be determined without further testing. I believe Dr. Matlock already discussed the possibility of endoscopy with you. Is that right?"

"He did. He explained the procedure already, and I'm ready to do whatever you suggest."

Rob stood up and retrieved an envelope from a large drawer in his desk, then pulled out Jack's UGI study. "I want to show you what's going on in your stomach." Placing the films on his radiology view box, he invited them closer for a better view. He then traced the outline of the stomach with his index finger, pointing out the area of deformity at the outlet of the stomach and the area of the pyloric valve, which regulates the flow of digesting food and liquids into the small intestine. "This valve, the pyloric valve, is becoming obstructed with an abnormal growth. By doing a biopsy with endoscopy, we should be able to get an exact diagnosis of the type of tumor. Now, unless another means of treatment is indicated by the biopsy, it's likely that you'll need an open operation to remove the obstruction so you can eat and function normally."

"Doc, I've already lost twelve pounds. Doc Matlock has me on a mainly liquid and soup diet. If you can fix that valve obstruction, I'll treat you to a steak dinner and see which one of us can eat the most."

Rob smiled. "That would be great, but let's get the procedures out of the way first and start you on the journey to recovery."

"Do you think you can remove whatever kind of tumor Jack has?" Janie asked.

He shrugged. "That depends again on the tissue type we get back from the biopsy. If it's something I feel comfortable with, I'll be glad to do the definitive surgery for you. If you prefer to go to a major medical center, I'll have no problem with that too. In fact, if you want me to, I'll make the referral for you now, including for the endoscopy, at another medical center."

"Won't be necessary. I trust you and Doc Matlock to do whatever's right for me. The two of you can take care of the whole thing. I got along fine with the hernia repair you did for me a few years ago."

Rob chuckled. "I'm glad for your vote of confidence, but if this is a serious type tumor, we'll both want the help and expertise of an oncologist."

Janie looked perplexed. "A what?"

Jack cleared his throat. "Lynn would understand what you mean, but I'm afraid you're over her mom and dad's heads."

"An oncologist is a specialist on diseases of the blood and of all kinds of tumors. We have an itinerant oncologist on staff, Dr. Gerald Stanberry. He has a clinic in our hospital once a week now. He comes from Methodist Hospital in Indianapolis, and many of our patients receive all their treatments here in Glen Falls."

"Sounds good to me, Doc," Jack said. "I'm not much on driving in Indianapolis. The traffic is terrible."

"Well, we'll help you make those decisions when the time comes. We all want whatever is best for you. Our goal is to see you recover your health." Glancing at Janie, Rob continued, "Now, I want no negative emotions. Whatever the diagnosis, we'll fight together to conquer this thing. Are we all on board?"

Jack and Janie nodded. "I just want to be told the entire truth when you know more about my disease," he said. "That's all I ask."

Rob patted Jack on the shoulder as the O'Conners sat back down. He handed them literature on the procedure and then stepped out into the hallway to have his nurse schedule upper endoscopy as soon as possible.

∿

THE NEXT MORNING, I made hospital rounds before office hours as usual. After seeing the last patient, I made my way to the surgical lounge to have my morning cup of coffee before going to the office. I also intended to check on Jack, whose endoscopy was scheduled at 8:00 a.m.

Soon, Dr. Hendrick joined me in the lounge area to give me an update on the results of the endoscopy. "Good morning, Carl." He pulled his mask down about his neck, poured a cup of coffee, sat down across from me, and shook his head. "It's not good news for Jack."

I took a deep breath, bracing myself. Jack was not only a patient but also a wonderful friend. He had pitched in when I remodeled my first office, and he advised his family and neighbors to see me for medical problems as he walked his mail rounds. Outgoing, cheerful, always a pleasant word as he left the mail each morning, always looking for ways to be helpful to me, to the office staff, and to my family—that was Jack.

Rob took a sip of his steaming black coffee before continuing. "Jack's still sedated. He was very apprehensive, and Bill Johnson had to give him a hefty dose of IV Valium with a little Morphine. He'll probably sleep for quite a while."

Forgetting all about my coffee, I nodded. "Not good, huh?"

He took another sip. "He has such a nice family. I got to know his daughter when she first came to observe, then worked in my office as a student. Always upbeat and excited to meet the patients."

Unable to speak, I nodded again.

"I took a biopsy of an ugly-appearing tumor that's nearly obstructing the pyloric valve and invading the mucosal wall. I sent it to the lab, and Fred Howard already looked at it under the microscope. He's a good pathologist, but I sure wish he was wrong." He took another sip of coffee, obviously hesitant to announce the dreadful news. "It's a poorly differentiated invasive adenocarcinoma involving the mucosa and at least the superficial muscle layer of the stomach."

I set my coffee on the table beside me. It had lost its appeal. "What's the next step?"

"When he wakes up, I'll have a discussion with him and his wife. Without surgery, he'll soon be obstructed by the tumor. He needs a resection to prevent complete obstruction, but the prognosis is poor, as you're aware."

I sighed and looked at the floor.

"His family is in the waiting room. Want to go with me to break the news?"

That was the least I could do. "Sure. As soon as you're ready."

◦～◦

JACK'S FAMILY awaited us in the lobby on the first floor. As we entered the area, Lynn noticed us and nudged her mother. Janie and William followed her as Rob and I led them to a quiet area where we could talk.

Rob sat across from Janie while I took a chair near Lynn and William. Rob's expression was serious, and Janie spoke in a small voice. "Reverend White stepped out for a moment. Can we wait for him to come back?"

He nodded. "Sure."

Seeing Reverend White approaching just then, I stood to shake his outstretched hand. "Good morning, Reverend. We were waiting on you." Turning to Rob, I said, "I believe you've met Dr. Hendrick."

Rob stood and smiled. "We've worked together often. I work on the body, and he works on the soul."

Reverend White smiled back and nodded but remained silent, probably noticing the expression on Janie's face. He took a seat beside her and patted her hand.

Rob took a deep breath, then exhaled slowly. "I'm afraid I don't have good news for you."

Tears filled Janie's eyes. William leaned over from her left, placing his arm around her shoulders. She looked small and vulnerable beside him. Lynn rose and stood behind her mother, placing both hands on her shoulders.

Rob continued, "First, your husband did well during the procedure. He's still sleeping off the medicine that Dr. Johnson gave him for the endoscopy. Unfortunately, Jack has gastric cancer, a gastric adenocarcinoma. It's a type that usually grows rapidly, invades, and spreads in the body."

Janie bowed her head as tears flowed freely. Reverend White sighed and looked away. William was trying to hide tears while Lynn covered her face, weeping softly.

Rob waited a few moments while the sad news penetrated, then said, "Folks, I didn't say there's no hope. I'm a firm believer in doing everything we can to help Jack as much as possible. He will need major

12

surgery to relieve the obstruction. We may even succeed in removing all the cancer, and the sooner the better. If nothing is done, it will spread and block his stomach, eventually resulting in death."

Janie looked up, blotting her eyes with a handkerchief that Lynn handed her. William nodded his thanks as I handed him a tissue. Lynn came around from behind her mother and sat down beside him.

"The encouraging news is that Jack's blood tests show no sign of distant spread. His liver and bone marrow blood tests are all normal. Maybe, just maybe, this tumor can be removed completely. There are more blood and x-ray tests that need to be run first, but he needs major surgery right away. All his preliminary tests prior to endoscopy looked good this morning."

Janie found her normal voice once more. "Will you do the surgery for Jack, Dr. Hendrick? He has a lot of faith in you."

"I'll be glad to if that is his wish, but I wouldn't have a problem in sending him to a major medical center if he prefers."

"You came from a large hospital practice to our little county hospital, didn't you?"

"Yes, four years ago, about the same time that Dr. Matlock began his practice. I wanted to raise my family in a smaller town than Indianapolis. That's why I'm here in Glen Falls."

She leaned forward. "Dr. Matlock has told us all about your expertise as a general surgeon. He has great faith in you, and we have faith in both of you."

Rob grinned. "I appreciate that, but I want to hear it from Jack before I do any more surgery. You understand that is only the first step. He must see our oncologist while he's recovering from surgery."

Janie cocked her head. "Who?"

Lynn reached across William to take her mother's left hand. "By a cancer specialist, Mom. Dr. Stanberry comes here at least weekly to see patients with cancer. He's an oncologist. I met him when I worked in Dr. Hendrick's office last summer. He's kind and very impressive. You'll like him."

Janie looked puzzled. "What will he do if the tumor is already removed?"

Rob nodded for me to explain, so I cleared my throat. "Even if the entire tumor is removed as far as we can determine by surgery, Dr. Stanberry can recommend steps to prevent it from coming back, such as chemotherapy or radiation, sometimes only one modality, sometimes both. He also follows patients who have had cancer, for several years following treatment. He sees them in our outpatient clinic in the hospital."

Janie furrowed her brows. "Okay, I think I understand, and that's good. When can we see Jack?"

Rob stood up. "As soon as he's more awake. The nurses will come and take you up to his room on the third floor. As long as he wants to have surgery here, we'll extend his admission. Once he's fully awake this afternoon, I'll return to have this talk again with Jack and any of you who want to be present. I'll schedule more tests for tomorrow, then surgery tentatively the following day."

Reverend White spoke up for the first time. "Can we all have a word of prayer for Jack before going our separate ways?"

Rob nodded. "Reverend, we have faith in you and in God, so go right ahead."

We bowed our heads, and Reverend White prayed for Jack, for the family, and for the physicians and nurses providing care. A spirit of sweetness and peace settled over us as he spoke in a reassuring voice with the One he had served so long, trusted completely, and knew so intimately.

Afterward, standing to depart for the office, I blinked away the moisture in my own eyes as I felt a measure of peace about Jack for the first time. It is comforting to be aware that there is a caring heavenly Father who intervenes in the affairs and lives of His children.

CHAPTER 3–NEVER A BORING MOMENT

$\mathcal{L}$ ate July and at 9:00 a.m., the sun already beat down on me as heat waves danced in the sultry air. I walked to the back of my office in Glen Oaks, mopped my forehead, unlocked the door, and hurried into the air-conditioned multipurpose room that served as medicine, lounge, and minor treatment area.

Donna looked up from the table, where she sat working on a stack of charts. "Good morning. What did Dr. Hendrick find on Jack's gastroscopy?"

"He found adenocarcinoma, at least stage 2, involving the superficial muscular layer of the stomach. It's not a large tumor, but it developed next to the pyloric valve and invaded the tissue causing a partial blockage."

Christine paused in the doorway leading to the hallway and outer office, cradling a cup of coffee in her hand. "What are his chances? I like that man and his family. Why does it have to happen to such a friendly person? Is Dr. Hendrick going to do more surgery? When is the operation?"

I mopped sweat from my forehead as I tried to decide where to start with Christine's rapid-fire interrogation. "It's sweltering out."

Christine cocked her head and placed her free hand on her hip. "Now, Doc, you haven't answered my question. I cannot work until I find out how Jack is doing."

I had to laugh. "Christine, which question do you want me to answer first? I believe you fired three or four at me."

"Okay, maybe I did. Please tell me what's going on."

Donna shook her head. "Get real. Why don't you be silent so he can answer you?"

Christine stuck her tongue out at her, then gave me a helpless look.

I chuckled again. "Okay, I'll try to satisfy your curiosity. Then will you go back to work?"

With an angelic smile, Christine curtsied. "Don't I always?"

"Jack has a tumor that will have to be resected to relieve the obstruction. That means at least a subtotal gastrectomy with a new connection to the second part of the small bowel, the jejunum. It's called a Billroth II. They remove the pyloric valve along with most of the lower or distal stomach while preserving part of the duodenum, the first part of the small intestine, as a blind sac in order not to disconnect the common bile duct which drains the liver, gallbladder, and pancreas. Confused yet?"

"Whew, you said it. But how is he doing? What's his chances?"

"The marvelous news is that we have found no sign of tumor elsewhere. There are no enlarged supraclavicular or epigastric lymph nodes. The liver functions and all other tests are normal so far."

"What kind of nodes did you say? What are they?"

"Stomach cancer can metastasize to regional lymph nodes, including those above the clavicles. Those are easy to palpate and are called supraclavicular nodes."

Christine came into the room and set down her coffee, then began checking her neck and supraclavicular areas.

Donna shook her head again. "Oh, brother. Christine, get a life."

Used to the playful banter, I continued, "Lymph nodes above the umbilicus also may contain metastatic disease. A nun named Sister Mary, as she cared for stomach cancer patients, discovered one. It's called Sister Mary's node."

Christine began rubbing her abdomen through her blouse.

I hastened to add, "That's an uncommon finding. We won't really know until after further tests and surgery. That will tell the story."

Donna stood. "Earth to Christine. Take your coffee and get to your desk. I think the phone is about to ring."

Christine gave her a mocking look. "I don't hear any phone ringing."

Donna scowled while brandishing a roll of paper towels. "Your head will ring and buzz in a minute after I bop you if you don't get to work. It's OB day, the rooms are full, and we have work to do. Understand?"

Christine saluted, pivoted, and made for the door, muttering under her breath, "Some people…"

I smiled as Donna handed me the first of seventeen charts. They were close friends who reveled in lighthearted banter. In a few hours, they would go to lunch together as if nothing had ever happened.

~

THE MORNING soon passed as I came to the last patient, Sally Christopher, twenty-nine years old with two children, ages three and four. I studied the chart before entering the room, noticing the normal vital signs and urinalysis. My only concern was a weight gain of six pounds in a week. She was now thirty-four weeks along and had been doing well.

Donna exited the room. "I'm worried about Sally," she whispered after closing the door. "She has a lot of swelling, and her abdomen is really growing. She complains of exhaustion and feeling terrible. The uterine fundus is already pushing up against her rib cage, and she looks exhausted."

"She's the last patient for the morning. Why don't you join us in the exam room? I may need your help."

Donna stepped in, took a seat, and picked up the youngest child while the four-year-old also clamored for attention. Grinning, she cradled one in each arm.

"Good morning, Sally," I said. "Donna tells me you're having a lot of swelling and discomfort. When did it start?"

Sally shrugged and shook her head. "I don't know for sure. This pregnancy is so much different from the other two. I had energy to spare and felt good when I carried Bennie and later Bobbie. Now, it's a major challenge to get out of bed in the morning. My abdomen is so heavy. My legs ache. I have constant heartburn. Something doesn't seem right."

I began by palpating her swollen abdomen, beginning at the fundus. "The baby's position is breech. I can outline the head right beneath your rib cage on your right side." Moving my hands down to the lower abdomen, attempting to outline the fetal pelvis, I paused, then repeated the examination. "I believe there is a head down here on your lower left side."

Sally gasped. "You aren't trying to tell me there are twins, are you?"

Hesitating, I positioned the fetoscope on my head. "I'm not sure of anything yet. Let me take a listen with this first."[1] I listened, focusing all my attention on the right upper abdomen for a few minutes before nodding at Sally. "Heartbeat good and strong at 156." I moved the fetoscope to the left lower abdomen and held up my hand for absolute silence as Donna quieted the children. I counted the heartbeat once, twice, then three times before announcing, "Heartbeat 120, strong and regular. But let me recheck." I must have moved the fetoscope up and down three times or more before pronouncing, "Two babies, one head-first and one breach. I can outline both of them by palpation and hear two distinct heartbeats, right where I would expect them to be."

Sally grimaced. "Oh no. Please tell me you're wrong."

I shook my head.

"I already have my hands full with two children. What am I going to do?"

I helped her sit back up on the cart and patted her on the shoulder. "You're a wonderful mom. I'm sure you'll be fine. Russell will be there to help you, and your sister lives right down the street with your folks. You will probably not go to full term. Twins most often come early."

She brushed aside a tear. "I'm sure you're right. I know I'll love them both. It's just such a shock."

Donna smiled, set the little ones in a chair together, and helped Sally down from the table. "I agree with Doc. You'll be fine, Sally. If you ever need help, I have the resumes of two young single ladies who would be happy to babysit for you."

"I'm sure I'll need help—often. Who do you have in mind?"

"Why, Christine and me. I look forward to it, and you know Christine."

Sally beamed. "You girls are so precious. I just love both of you, and I believe you mean it."

Christine pushed the door open a crack. "We sure do. How wonderful. How exciting! I can't wait for them to get here."

I shook my head in dismay at her eavesdropping, but we all enjoyed a laugh together.

~

DONNA AND CHRISTINE prepared to go to the House Pharmacy and General Store for lunch. Ethel House served wonderful lunches, aided by her daughters. Just before locking the door, Christine turned to me. "I almost forgot. Dr. Hendrick's office called to tell you that Dr. Stanberry will see Jack in the morning. If everything turns out okay, Dr. Hendrick plans to operate the next day, this Thursday. I sure hope he finds no more cancer. Tell him we're praying for his recovery."

Donna nodded. "Yes, please do."

I retrieved my ham and cheese sandwich and Diet Coke from the refrigerator. As I sat gazing out the back windows of the office, munching on my sandwich, watching our neighbor's horses grazing in the pasture behind my office, a sense of peace and rest permeated my mind. I realized just how much I loved this town and the people who lived here.

CHAPTER 4—DAY OF SURGERY

*T*hursday morning found me en route to the hospital, driving the back roads through the countryside, windows rolled down to enjoy the cool freshness of the early morning air. The local radio station promised a warm day with lots of sunshine after the overcast sky cleared.

Preoccupied and troubled about what would be found during Jack O'Connor's surgery, I arrived at a four-way stop. A meadowlark heralded the morning from a corner fencepost while house sparrows twittered in the bushes beside a whitewashed farmhouse, and the pastoral scene suddenly illuminated with dazzling light as the sun broke through the dark clouds. Reassured that Jack had placed his confidence in God, my spirits lifted a little.

I proceeded on toward Glen Falls, passing cornfields, lush pasture lands with grazing Hereford and Angus cattle, and farm lots with neat red barns, tall brick or concrete silos, and large corrugated steel grain bins. A sense of peace and calmness gradually permeated my being. Inhaling deeply, I savored the scent of new-mown hay as farm tractors rolled through the fields. The farm life and beautiful landscape I saw by avoiding morning rush-hour traffic on the interstate refreshed my soul, and the extra time spent on the slower drive cleared my mind and thinking for the day ahead. Grasping for increased faith, I sent a prayer heavenward for my friend and patient, Jack O'Connor.

I arrived at the hospital around 7:00 a.m., parked in the doctors' lot, and made my way to the side entrance. Robins sang exuberantly in the giant old oak tree on the hospital grounds. Anxious yet filled with hope, I flipped on my light switch, notifying the hospital operator that I was now in the house. With surgery scheduled at 7:30 a.m., I hurried to the third floor for one more brief visit with Jack.

∽

JACK'S ROOM was filled to capacity with his wife, children, and several other members of his large extended family. Reverend White and his wife were there to encourage the family and be with them during the surgical procedure.

"Good morning, everyone," I said. "How are you, Jack? All set?"

"Yeah, Doc. I think you know most of my family. I have many people rooting for me."

"Has Dr. Hendrick been in already?"

Jack grinned. "Yeah, he beat you here by at least a half hour. You must be slipping."

I smiled and nodded. He needed the lighthearted banter. "I guess you noticed my late arrival."

"Will you be in surgery with Doctor Hendrick?" Janie asked.

"I sure will. I'll be assisting him. We'll see the family in the lobby afterward. But in the meantime, I'll see you in the OR in a few minutes, Jack."

Jack managed a tight smile. "I'll be there. Make sure he only takes out what he's supposed to."

∽

MASKED, scrubbed, gloved, and gowned, I stood directly across from Rob Hendrick as we awaited the signal from Bill Johnson, a family doctor and anesthesiologist, to begin the operation. Finally satisfied, Bill nodded and said, "He's ready. You can cut now."

Candy Benton, surgical scrub nurse on Rob's right side, handed him a scalpel. Surgical towels and a special surgical sheet had already been applied to Jack's abdomen following the initial scrubbing with Betadine surgical soap.

Rob deftly made a vertical incision in the exposed epigastric area. After entering the abdominal cavity, he did a rapid survey of the organs both visually and by palpation to rule out any obvious extension of the cancer to other organs. Afterward, he glanced over the top of his glasses and nodded. "So far so good. There doesn't appear to be any seeding of the cancer throughout the peritoneum." Turning toward Bill Johnson, he continued, "I'm proceeding with a subtotal gastrectomy and Billroth II anastomosis. We'll be here a little while."

"Go right ahead," Bill answered. "He's doing fine. Vital signs all stable."

The distal stomach with the pyloric valve and a segment of the duodenum, the first part of the small intestine, required excision first. Further exploration of the abdominal cavity revealed several regional lymph nodes that Rob removed and sent for evaluation to the pathologist, Fred Howard. Although two out of fifteen lymph nodes removed revealed adenocarcinoma, the rest were completely negative with no extension of tumor through the wall of the stomach beyond the inner superficial muscular layer.

About two hours later, I relaxed in the surgery lounge area with a cup of coffee while Rob dictated the surgical op note and Jack rested in the recovery room for careful monitoring while anesthesia wore off. We checked on Jack once more, then proceeded to the lobby to advise the family and friends of the outcome.

～

AFTER WE HAD everyone gathered in a corner of the lobby where there was some privacy for the group, Rob took the initial lead in the discussion. "Jack is in recovery now, and he is doing very well as far as surgical concerns. We had no significant or excessive blood loss. His vital signs remained stable throughout the operation, and we removed all the cancer we could find. The cancer in the stomach itself was limited pretty much to what we saw on x-ray and at biopsy. It did not erode through the wall of the stomach into the abdominal cavity. Unfortunately, there were two positive lymph nodes with cancerous tissue present. We removed those. Thirteen other lymph nodes were negative for cancer cells. With this type of stomach cancer, it is usually extremely aggressive, so we must've caught it early. Almost without exception, in the past when I've operated on similar cases, it's usually already widespread. Not so in this case, and that is tremendous news." Pausing, he cleared his throat. "Questions?"

Janie appeared both relieved and concerned. "Does that mean you got all the cancer?"

"We hope so, but we can't be one hundred percent sure," Rob responded. "There could be microscopically small cancer cells still present. That's why we asked Dr. Stanberry to see your husband. He will determine the next steps in therapy, which we hope will be just preventive with no return of the cancer."

Lynn gave her mother a hug. "That sure sounds better than what I expected." She lowered her gaze to the floor. "I know it wasn't a good idea, but I spent over two hours in the medical library at the university yesterday, reading about stomach cancer. From what I learned, I came here today with no hope at all." She looked up at us. "At least Daddy has a fighting chance."

Rob smiled. "Well, I have another major case scheduled in just a few minutes. If you'll excuse me, I'm sure Dr. Matlock will be glad to continue addressing your concerns. I'll see your husband back in the room later this afternoon when all my other surgeries are completed. If there are other questions you need to discuss with me, I'll be available for you."

William stepped forward to shake hands with me. "Thanks for being there for Dad, and for Mom too. This has been a genuine shock to all of us."

"You're welcome. Do you have any more questions for me?"

"Will we be able to see him soon?" Reverend White asked. "I don't want to go home until I've seen Jack again. I want to pray with him after he wakes up."

"I'd say it'll probably be another hour, perhaps longer. It was a major operation, so it'll be a little while before he's stable enough to go back to his room."

Visibly relieved, the group broke up. Two of Jack's brothers stopped to shake hands and express appreciation. As the others left, Lynn had a few more questions. "Do you have any idea how long it will be before Daddy can have any treatment, chemotherapy or radiation?"

"That'll be up to Dr. Stanberry and Dr. Hendrick. I would say it'll be somewhere between four and six weeks before it'll be safe to proceed with further treatment. His wounds will have to heal first. He'll also need to be taking food and having normal bowel function again. Whether there will be chemotherapy, radiation, or some combination of both, that will be up to Dr. Stanberry."

Janie reached for my hand. "Thanks so much, Doctor. We appreciate all you do for us. Be sure to thank Christine and Donna too. Christine called last night right after your office hours to tell me she and Donna were praying for us. They will never know how much that means to our family. They're such sweet ladies."

"I will convey that message to them. They really care about people. Being patient advocates is a concern they do not take lightly. The girls don't just work for me but for all the patients and families in our practice, and will appreciate your kind comments."

~

AFTER FINISHING patient rounds later that morning, I left the hospital for my usual scenic ride back to the office, thankful and hopeful that Jack O'Conner would survive this potentially aggressive cancer.

CHAPTER 5—FEAR AND UNCERTAINTY

*E*ntering through the back door of my office, I immediately felt something amiss. I checked my watch and noted the time, 1:30 p.m., before realizing that the very quietness of the office constituted what differed about my usual entrance. Today, there was no steady stream of conversation, no one to question me about the surgery, no buzzing chatter from the outer office. Puzzled, I placed my medical bag on the table and then opened the door to the waiting room/reception area.

No wonder quiet reigned supreme. Not one patient had arrived. Donna had her back to me, busily arranging magazines in the rack across the room and tidying up the area. Christine sat at her desk just around the corner, with a view of the entire spacious waiting area but with her head down as she took a bite out of a sandwich.

I cleared my throat and shut the door behind me.

Donna jumped about a foot in the air, and Christine gave an ear-shattering scream as she nearly knocked over her chair in fright. Donna wheeled about with her hand over her heart as Christine charged out of the reception area racing for the front door and safety. She had the door open, preparing to exit, when Donna began laughing.

"We didn't hear you come in," Donna said. "We've been so worried about Jack and his family. I think this is the third time I've straightened and dusted the waiting room today. Christine has all but driven me mad with her gloomy projections. She's been drumming on the desk with her fingers and proclaiming doomsday scenarios."

Christine closed the door with a dour expression and a *humph*. She faced me with her hands on her hips. "Doc, you just took ten years from me. I've never been so scared in all my life."

I did my best to look sorry, but Donna's laughing and pointing at Christine proved my undoing. My shoulders shook as I gave up all pretense of seriousness and laughed with abandon as I sat down on a chair across from the front door.

Donna collapsed in a chair by the magazine rack, also laughing.

Christine looked at us with a raised right eyebrow. "Okay, you two comedians, what's so funny?"

Donna found her voice before I did. "Just go look in the mirror, you silly goose. Then you'll know why we're laughing."

Christine frowned, rushed from the waiting room, and fled down the hallway to the restroom as we continued to enjoy her discomfiture. Soon, we heard a yell from the restroom. "Oh, you terrible sadists! What's so funny to laugh at a poor working girl who just ruined her best blouse. And with patients scheduled to arrive at two fifteen, whatever am I going to do?"

Donna got up, still laughing, and went to help Christine clean up the damage. Within five minutes, both returned to the waiting room where I had finally composed myself.

Christine continued to sadly wipe at the ketchup stains on her other-wise-stylish light-blue blouse. She cast an accusing eye my way. "You could at least let a girl suffer in quiet dignity."

I smiled. "You're right. We shouldn't have laughed."

Donna smirked. "You would've laughed at either of us and you know it."

For several seconds, Christine stood looking down at the stain.

Finally, a smile flickered across her face. "I bet I looked a sight." With that, her irrepressible good humor took over as she chuckled about her situation. "The patients will think one of you stabbed me. That's what I will tell them. It'll be all over town by quitting time today."

Donna rolled her eyes. "Some people will do anything for attention."

She smiled. "You bet. Now please help me clean up the mess at my desk. I believe I threw the rest of my sandwich on top of the stack of charts. They're 'bleeding' too."

"I'm sorry I scared you, but I thought we were to start at one thirty today. I was on time, but I couldn't believe the stillness from the outer office."

"We figured you'd be a little late as usual," Christine said, "and the first two patients rescheduled for next week anyway. Besides all that, we want to know about Jack. How is he? Has the cancer spread? Did you get all of it out? How's his family doing? They're some of my favorite people. I miss Jack handing in the mail every morning. Will he need chemotherapy and radiation?"

I winked at Donna, who stood behind Christine flapping the fingers of her right hand up and down on her thumb, trying to keep up with the rapid-fire speech. "Our girl's back to normal, that's for sure."

Christine smiled and did her usual curtsy. "Well, are you going to fill us in or not?"

I glanced at my watch. "Sure. I'll give you what details I can as you straighten up your desk. We have about twenty minutes before the first patient is due, and the aroma from that smashed hamburger on top of the charts is about to make me hungry again. Please do something with it."

I stood outside the smaller reception room at the open top of the French door to fill in the details as the ladies removed most of the evidence of the destroyed lunch. "Well, first, Dr. Hendrick removed all the visible cancer and several regional lymph nodes. Unfortunately, two of the nodes were positive for cancer cells, so it's likely that we didn't get everything."

Christine teared up at the news. "Will he live long?"

"I really don't know, but the good news is that thirteen out of fifteen lymph nodes had no cancer cells. Also, the cancer invaded the muscle wall of the pyloric valve and the superficial wall of the stomach muscle, but strangely enough, it didn't penetrate any deeper, and that's a promising sign. It's possible that he may live several years with good care and follow-up with oncology. As to the treatment, Dr. Stanberry will decide. Chemotherapy is likely, but I don't know about radiation. The underlying organs like the pancreas are easily damaged with radiation treatment for cancer of the stomach. It'll be up to his best judgment what to do next. Regarding the O'Conner family, they're doing as well as one might expect with such a life-threatening disease facing Jack."

Donna sighed. "Is it usual for stomach carcinoma not to be widespread at initial surgery?"

"No. Stomach cancer frequently doesn't give enough warning signs. The patients I helped care for during my training frequently had widespread disease obvious on entry to the peritoneal cavity during the exploratory procedure."

Donna nodded. "I've seen cases like that in training too. With our current technology, small peritoneal implants of cancer can go undetected until surgery."

"That's exactly right. Someday we'll likely have improved technology, but for now we look for cancer that has metastasized to large organs like the liver or lungs. If none is there, exploratory surgery sometimes finds widespread cancer in the abdomen anyway. I repeat, the improved prognosis for Jack is that he had no other evidence of metastatic cancer."

A car pulled up in front of the office.

Donna opened a cabinet drawer, pulled out a folded red sweater, and thrust it at Christine. "Here, put this on over your blouse. No one will ever know about the stain."

"Bright red and light blue!" Christine shrieked. "I'd rather they see the stain. Besides, it's summer. A sweater looks as weird as the stain. Forget it."

Donna wagged her finger at her. "Don't ever say I didn't try to help."

Christine stuck her tongue out. "Such help. I'll do better without your assistance, thank you very much."

As I began walking toward the break room, Christine called out, "I forgot to tell you. Lynn O'Conner is a work-in after the scheduled appointments. She wants to talk with you about her dad. She sounded very concerned over the phone. Doesn't want her mom to know she's coming in to see you. Now you're forewarned."

~

THE REST of the afternoon proceeded normally with a few summer viral colds and gastroenteritis cases mixed in with routine physicals for school children since the fall semester would begin in a little over a month. There were no serious problems, for which I was grateful after the stress of major cancer surgery. I finished the day at 6:05 p.m., only a little over an hour after closing time.

Christine met me in the hallway as I exited the last exam room. "Lynn just called. She's running a little late."

"How late?"

"Only an hour or so. I told her we'd wait until she gets here, probably around seven."

"You told her we'd wait an hour or more for her to get here?" I tried not to let irritation edge into my voice.

She nodded innocently.

"Christine, I have a date to take my wife and children out to eat this evening, a rare-enough event as it is. I can't wait that long. By the time we finish, the better restaurants in Glen Falls will all be closed."

Christine beamed. "You can relax, she'll be here in five minutes. I just wanted to get even with you and Donna for laughing mercilessly at me this afternoon. You should have heard Donna go off when I told her how late she has to stay. Don't say anything, please. She's still fuming. I didn't tell her any different yet."

I took a deep breath. "I should have known what you were up to. By the way, what did the patients say about your soiled blouse?"

"You'll find that equally amusing. You know Laura Dawson, right?"

I nodded. "You mean our sweet little old town gossip, I presume."

She grinned from ear to ear. "The very one and only. Well, she came in to pick up the prescription you refilled for her blood pressure today, and being very observant, she naturally noticed the unsightly stains on my beautiful blouse."

"Oh, naturally. Not much gets by her."

Christine clasped her hands together over her head like she had just been declared a champion. "I told her you made me drop my sandwich, which ruined my blouse. Then you and Donna laughed at me. Donna didn't hear me tell her about what happened, but she walked into the reception office just before Laura left."

"And?"

"Laura scolded Donna for mistreating me and slammed the door as she left in a huff. It was so delicious. Donna turned to me in confusion and wanted to know why Laura acted so hateful."

"No way!"

Christine nodded. "By now, Laura has spread it all over town that you and Donna threw food at me and ruined a perfectly good blouse."

"Surely not."

"Oh, yes. Donna called in two prescriptions for Barry House to fill, and he wanted to know why you two were throwing food at me."

I gasped. "You didn't tell her that, did you?"

"Of course not. I may be a prankster, but I'm not malicious. Laura didn't have her hearing aids in today, and you know how dangerous that is. Anyway, Barry didn't believe her. He just thought it was outrageously funny. He asked me to give you a hard time over it."

As Christine walked back to the outer office, I muttered to myself, "Small towns. No secrets. Never."

She stopped and looked over her shoulder. "What's that?"

"Nothing important. You've just got me talking to myself now. We'll live this down. Fortunately, few believe anything Laura Dawson has to say."

Christine hurried on down the hallway, calling, "Got to hurry. I think I just heard Lynn come in the front door. I'll tell Donna the truth, but she still won't appreciate my prank. No sense of humor at all."

~

LYNN O'CONNER SAT on the edge of a leather chair across from me in my office, hands tightly clasped, golden hair falling about her shoulders, and deep brown eyes glistening with tears she fought to hold back.

Donna, standing quietly by her chair, offered her a Kleenex.

Lynn nodded her thanks and dabbed at her eyes.

Donna leaned down and hugged her. "Shall I leave? I'll be glad to if you prefer speaking with the doctor alone."

Lynn shook her head. "I don't mind if you stay. You already know what's going on in my life. I appreciate your concern so very much."

I sat back in my chair, folded my hands, and nodded for Lynn to begin.

She dried her tears and clenched the tissue in her right hand. "I'm so worried about Daddy. I've spent hours in the medical library reading everything I can find about gastric carcinoma, and the news isn't good."

"I know. I'm so sorry. I'm glad that in times like these we have the Great Physician to turn to in our need. You still believe that, don't you, Lynn?"

She considered that and finally shrugged. "I'm a little mixed up about God and the Bible right now. Why would God allow my wonderful father to suffer such a terrible fate? Most of my professors don't even believe in God or a higher power."

"I understand. I faced the same skepticism from many of my teachers in college and medical school." I took a deep breath. "What helped me through that was the faith of my parents. They have always been a great inspiration to me. I watched their consistent lives in the good times and in the bad ones. They always lived out their faith regardless of the personal cost. And sometimes it cost them a lot. No amount of so-called scientific reasoning can ever talk me out of the reality of Christian lives I've witnessed."

Lynn looked up and nodded slightly.

"If I know your parents as I think I do, you also have the same vital Christian witness in their lives. Isn't that so?"

"Yes. My parents have always set a godly example for my brother and me." She bowed her head. "I guess I'm not a very strong Christian, but this has me reeling."

"Having doubt is not a sign of weakness or sin. After all is said and done, we still belong to the frail human race. God allowed sin and suffering to enter the world because we live in a fallen world, not the one He originally planned."

"You sound just like Daddy. He told me something like that before surgery. I know he's worried but not nearly as much as I am."

I waited as she cleared her throat and wiped her eyes again. "Your father is a good Christian man. He has faith in Dr. Hendrick and the oncologist, but he also trusts Jesus to care for him."

"I know, and that helps me. But I also want your advice. I just finished a summer school course in pharmacology and am to begin my third year in pre-med in September. I've been told that if I do well, I can get into med school after three years. My first year of med school would count as my fourth year in college."

"That's right. Students can do that by keeping their grades up and passing the MCAT, the medical college admission test, with a satisfactory score. I believe you can do it. I hope you try for that option."

Lynn shook her head slowly, her face unusually pale and pinched. "That's what I want to do, but with Daddy ill, I don't know where the money will come from to even finish college."

I leaned back in my chair, gazing at my medical school diploma and family practice board certification hanging on the opposite wall as I pondered the situation. I nodded toward them. "Do you see those certificates?"

Lynn sighed. "Yes. That's what I'd hoped for so much. You and these ladies have been my inspiration to succeed in medicine."

"I earned those certificates in various ways," I said. "My dad helped me as much as he could. I worked during my summers off, and I had some school loans along with a scholarship I won for college. Where there's a will, there's a way, as the old saying goes."

"I know, but…"

I held up my hands. "Actually, I just know of a scholarship the hospital is offering to a promising student, medical or nursing, who agrees to return and practice in the community for at least three years."

"Really?"

"Really. I also know the members of the committee who will decide on the award."

Lynn smiled for the first time. "So you think I might have a chance?"

"If I know the members as I think I do, you'll win the scholarship with no real contest."

"Oh, if only I could. That would make Daddy happy too. I just told him I was thinking about dropping out of school for now. I didn't realize he would be so distressed. I think he was blaming himself."

"When you see him this evening, tell him you're not giving up. A wealthy anonymous benefactor of the hospital has already made suffi-cient funds available for a student to attend college and medical or nursing school as long as two requirements are met: academic achieve-ment and proven need of financial assistance. I have no doubt you'll qualify. In fact, there are already sufficient funds available for two students per year for the next five years. I happen to have an application here in my desk." I pulled it out and handed it to her. "Go home and fill it out. You can turn it in at the human resources office or bring it back to me to turn in, but do it right away."

"You really think I might qualify?"

"Your proud parents already told me about your 4.0 average for the first two years of college. I trust they weren't stretching the truth."

Lynn blushed. "They weren't."

"Then it's time for you to stop worrying. Reclaim your faith in God for the future and for your father's recovery. It's true he has a worrisome type of cancer, but it's also very early in development compared to what we usually find at initial surgery."

Lynn stood up and shook my hand. "Thanks for giving me hope and a plan. I'll do my best to keep my faith intact."

Donna walked her to the waiting room as I turned to finish her chart.

Preparing to leave, Lynn asked, "Do you know who is on the scholarship committee at the hospital?"

Donna beamed. "I know some members. Dr. Matlock and Dr. Hendrick are two of them. I believe they carry a lot of weight on the committee."

"Oh?" She grinned in delight before a look of consternation came over her countenance. "I wouldn't want them to favor me over a more deserving candidate."

"Don't worry about that, Lynn," Christine said from where she sat at her desk. "He already knows who the other candidates are, and he won't cheat. If he says you are likely to get the award, well, that's where I'm putting my money."

Donna nodded. "That's right. Be sure and fill out the paperwork and get it in as soon as you can. Before you came in, he told me that the deadline is in one week. He asked me to be sure you know that."

"You all discussed this before I came in?"

"You didn't think Doc came up with this plan all by his lonesome, did you?" Christine said.

Donna laughed. "Christine, you're impossible. It's mostly Doc's idea. You have just been harassing him about it for a couple of days."

Lynn smiled and heaved a sigh of relief. "You girls! Well, what do I owe you today?"

Christine grinned. "Doc says it's on the house. He marked your bill as 'consultation, no charge.'"

"Tell him,"—Lynn's voice caught—"tell him thanks so much. And thank you, ladies, for being such precious friends."

Donna patted her shoulder. "Keep your chin up and know that we're praying for you and your dad."

Christine nodded. "Ditto that. Now go fill out those papers. I'll bug you until you do."

Donna raised her eyebrows. "She will for sure. Better fill them out."

CHAPTER 6—NEW LIFE

our days later, I joined Rob Hendrick for a cup of coffee in the hospital doctors' lounge prior to early morning rounds. "Good morning." As I filled my cup, I glanced at him. "It's a beautiful sunny day that promises to be another hot one. I'm about ready for fall weather."

He looked up from the morning edition of the *Glen Falls Daily* and smiled. "I'm ready for cooler weather too, but time already passes too quickly as I grow older. I'm in no hurry."

I took a seat in a comfortable leather lounge chair across from Rob, setting my coffee on the mahogany end table beside me to let it cool a little. "Have you seen Jack O'Conner yet?"

"Not this morning, but I visited him about eight o'clock last night when I was called to the ER to see a patient with abdominal pain. That patient had gastroenteritis, not a surgical emergency, but I don't blame the ER doc. The family demanded another opinion. I guess they think we have nothing else to do with our time off."

I nodded, knowing the feeling quite well.

"At any rate, Jack seems to be doing fine. I talked with Gerald Stanberry yesterday. Jack can start chemotherapy in about six weeks as long as he continues to make excellent progress." Rob frowned. "I feel uneasy about Jack, though. He seems almost too cheerful. I don't know if he's in denial or just attempting to live out his faith. I talked with him again about the need for aggressive treatment as soon as possible. He just smiled and told me he was certain everything will be all right. He almost seems to have a mental disconnect regarding his diagnosis and prognosis. Do you think he's emotionally stable?"

I considered that. "I think so. He's usually optimistic about life. I'll try to sound him out when I see him this morning. I hope he's not in serious denial. That won't help him face the ordeal of chemotherapy."

Rob drained his cup before standing and offering me the newspaper. "Not much in it. Only the local gossip, police and ambulance runs, hospital admissions and discharges, the usual."

As I reached for the paper, the overhead intercom came on with a pop. "Dr. Matlock, OB stat. Dr. Matlock, OB stat."

Leaving my coffee, I jumped up. "Guess I don't have time now."

I ran up the nearby stairway two steps at a time to the OB department on the third floor. Flying to the nurses' station, where OB medical assistant Sharon Cunningham consoled Russell Christopher, I stopped long enough to ask, "Sally?"

She nodded her head. "She just got here and is already dilated 9 cm and in hard labor. She said you recently diagnosed twins, and she's early. I think you have time to change into scrubs, but you'd better hurry."

"Right. Excuse me, Russell. Got to get ready. Do you want to go with us to the delivery room?"

Russell collapsed into a chair that Sharon scooted beneath him in a timely fashion. Pale and sweaty, he shook his head. "Sorry, I can't do it. Can't stand the sight of blood."

Sharon called after me, "I have to stay here with him, but you'll have expert help today. We just finished morning report and Mrs. Long is still here from the night shift. She and the day shift charge nurse, Mrs. Jarret, are both back in the delivery room."

I CHARGED INTO THE DOCTORS' dressing room, changed in record time, and rushed to the door of the delivery room as I tied my mask and surgical cap in place. Stopping by the large enamel sink outside the door, I surveyed the activity. "Do I have time to scrub?"

Mrs. Jarret—tall, trim, methodical, and unperturbed—stood at Sally's right side starting an IV. Mrs. Long—short, plump, jolly, and laid back—glanced over her mask at me as she got Sally into position for delivery. "If you hurry. I don't see a head yet."

"Everything's fine," Mrs. Jarret added. "The first baby is definitely cephalic. I barely had time to do a quick exam in the labor room. I'm not sure, but I think number two is breech. I have the Piper forceps ready for you. I got the IV in place, so we're about ready. Her membranes ruptured on the way into delivery."

I scrubbed quickly and hurried into the room as Mrs. Long adjusted the overhead lights and Mrs. Jarret pumped up the delivery table with the foot pedal on her side. Mrs. Long helped me into the sterile blue gown and disposable sterile rubber gloves. I turned around in time to deliver Baby A, making sure the head came out in a controlled manner. I suctioned out the nares, noticed a brief attempt at respiratory effort, guided the delivery of the wet slippery body, and rubbed her back with my knuckles until she arched away from my hand with loud squalls of protest. After clamping and cutting the cord, I handed the infant to Mrs. Long. "Baby A, girl. Born at 7:20 a.m. Now for Baby B."

I did a rapid internal examination and glanced up at Sally. She continued to moan and push, straining forcefully to expel Baby B. "You're doing a great job. There is a separate amniotic sac, probably fraternal, non-identical twin, but we'll soon know."

From the tray beside me I grabbed the syringe with the trumpet-type grip for the plunger. "I'll rupture the membranes in a second, but the second baby is definitely breech. I'll likely need to use forceps to deliver

40

the head, and I'll make an incision to expedite delivery. That's the episiotomy incision we discussed in the office."

Sally nodded, her face turning shades of purple as she grunted, trying to expel the baby. "Hurry! Get it out."

"Okay, this will sting for a second." I injected 1% lidocaine in the perineum and made a left mediolateral incision to allow for the increased space usually necessary in a breech delivery. Next, I took a clamp with sharp edges, reached past the still protruding cord Baby A left behind, and ruptured the membranes of the second infant. Amniotic fluid rushed out as I stepped aside, and two tiny legs slid down into the pelvis. I grasped the legs and found the position to be posterior, facing toward the floor. Once sure the second cord wasn't compressed by the baby's body, I allowed Baby B to deliver to the mid-trunk spontaneously.

Sally pushed herself up on her elbows to get more leverage, her face still purple with pushing, and I noted a few petechiae forming around her forehead and cheeks as she strained. I needed to get this baby out. If the small blood vessels in the face were rupturing from her tremendous efforts at expulsion, I could only imagine what might happen should a larger blood vessel burst internally.

Mrs. Long anticipated my next move and handed me a sterile towel to wrap around the tiny body. Then she took the towel from me, providing support for the baby, as I gently rotated the little body back and forth, reached up to grasp the elbows, straightened the little arms, and pulled them down one at a time to free up the shoulders.

I glanced over at Mrs. Jarret, who wiped amniotic fluid from Baby A as she continued to protest with offended cries of outrage. Our new overhead radiant warmer was working out fine. Mrs. Jarret nodded and smiled from behind her mask. "Baby A looks fine. She's a keeper. One-minute Apgar score 10, if you agree."

"Certainly. She looks great. Now to get this one the rest of the way out." I picked up the Piper forceps, especially designed for delivering the head in breech births, and reached down to place the forceps from beneath the infant. Quickly assuring myself that the placement was correct, I pulled downward first, followed by an upward arc of traction, gently applied, and slowly delivered the head. Although the procedure looked barbaric, a breech baby delivered this way was actually safer from head trauma than a baby allowed to be battered on the perineum during the birth process. (In those days, breech babies were not routinely sent to C-section.)

Mrs. Long continued to support the baby with the towel as I eased the head out with another last gush of residual amniotic fluid. This time I couldn't get out of the way, and fluid and blood from the delivery soiled my sterile gown. The nurse handed me Baby B still wrapped in a sterile blue towel. I removed the towel, cut the cord, suctioned out the nares, and gently stimulated him until a loud shriek rent the air as the little fella vociferously protested bright lights, loud voices, and giant tormenters after leaving the cozy warm darkness of the womb.

Normally, Pitocin 10 mg is given with delivery of the shoulders, but with a breech delivery, I had to wait for the second infant's birth. The Pitocin acted as a stimulant to contract the uterus, and the last thing I wanted was two trapped placentas with continued bleeding.

Sally allowed her head to fall back down on the cart, relieved of her burden yet too weak to hold either baby, so I held up the last precious child for her to see. "Baby B. B for boy, born at 7:35."

Sally managed a brief smile. "Wonderful. It was hard, but they're worth it. Now I have three boys and finally a baby girl. I'm ready to quit. I need to have the surgeon fix me before I go home. I can't go through this again."

Glancing back down, I saw that the first cord had slid much farther out. I gave a slight tug, and the placenta with residual cord slid into the basin I held to catch it. I inspected the placenta for completeness and laid it aside for later inspection by our pathologist. The second placenta soon delivered in similar fashion, and I nodded at Mrs. Jarret. "Pitocin 10 mg IM now."

I did a bimanual exam to exclude inadvertently retained tissue, massaging the uterus between my right hand positioned in the vaginal canal and my left hand placed on the lower abdominal wall to encourage uterine contraction and prevent excessive bleeding.

Sally Christopher had done an amazing job.

～

AFTER CHANGING into a fresh set of scrubs, I searched for Russell Christopher. At the desk, Sharon motioned to me. "If you're looking for Mr. Christopher, I sent him back to the main lobby downstairs. He was rocking back and forth like he was the one in labor. I didn't have time to watch him. When his brother showed up, I asked him to take Russell downstairs and get him something to drink."

"Okay. I'll look for him in the lobby after I dictate a delivery note."

I smiled. Russell had never had much of a stomach for blood or trauma. He had been one of the first people to faint in my office, overcome by the sight of blood after he cut his finger at work. That had been a hectic day that I wouldn't soon forget. Interesting. Russell was a big, powerful man who had no problem facing most of life's problems otherwise.

～

RUSSELL SAT in a corner of the lobby sipping a coke while his brother, Josh, kept him company. He still had a sick, pasty appearance that only worsened when he saw me coming. He managed to stand, weaving unsteadily on his feet. "Are we all done?" He hesitated, trying to collect his thoughts. "I mean, did Sally have the babies? Everything okay?"

"You have a healthy set of twins, a little girl weighing in at 5 lb. 7 oz and a boy weighing 5 lb. 12 oz. That's a lot of babies for a little woman, but your wife did very well. Both babies appear healthy. Their birth scores were great, and their initial exams are normal."

Russell mopped his forehead with a handkerchief and grunted as if in pain. "I better set back down for a minute. Don't feel so good right now."

"Are you ill?"

Josh winked as he helped Russell back to his seat.

Russell sat down, cradling his head in his hands as he slumped over on the couch. Josh cupped his hands and whispered, "He's always been queasy around hospitals. I'm surprised he got here on his own without me. He'll be okay. I'll take him up to see the clan when he settles down."

"Okay, Josh. Great to see you. Take care of Russell. Sally and the babies are fine."

Josh grinned. "Sure, Doc. Will do. Not to worry."

I pivoted about to continue hospital rounds. Now for Jack.

Josh called after me, "Say, Doc. When Russell feels better, will it be okay for me to take him up to tell his Uncle Jack about the babies?"

I wheeled back around. "I didn't know Jack is related to you fellas."

Russell nodded as Josh continued, "Actually, he's Sally's uncle, but the three of us are fishing buddies. He's only Russell's uncle by marriage, but Jack is like family to both of us. You should know by now that everyone is related to everyone else in Glen Oaks."

I smiled. "I didn't know about the relationship, but sure. It'll be good for Jack. Please give me a few minutes to visit with him first." I nodded at Russell. "And be sure he's up to it before you take him up to the surgery floor."

Josh beamed. "Of course. I don't want to pick this big ox up off the floor. I'll be sure he's back to normal first. He'll be A-OK in a half hour or so."

CHAPTER 7—UNCERTAIN FUTURE

*A*fter perusing Jack's chart with the latest lab results and recent vital signs, I poked to his room considering my opening words. With a heavy heart, mustering courage, I entered room 306 with a feigned confident cheerfulness and a beaming smile. "Good morning. How are you feeling today?"

Jack sat beside his bed in a comfortable chair reading the morning newspaper while sipping a cup of coffee. He wore the usual hospital gown tied in back at the neck and waist. An IV continued to drip at a reduced rate in his left mid-forearm.

He gave his usual warm smile as he laid his paper aside on the bed. "I'm doing wonderful, as always."

I pulled up a chair nearby. He couldn't really be that optimistic. I cleared my throat and began carefully. "I understand you saw Dr. Stanberry yesterday regarding chemotherapy."

"Sure did. He's a likeable fellow. Open, frank, and very trustworthy."

He had to be in denial. "Did you discuss the medications, side effects, and prognosis?"

Jack held up his right hand. "Hold on, Doc. You fellas ask too many questions at once."

I chuckled. "You're right. My mistake. Guess I'm in too much of a hurry."

"You can say that again." He joined me in chuckling. "What do you want to know first?"

"Let's start with chemotherapy."

"That's more like it. And I have a straightforward answer. I didn't understand a thing he said except that I would likely be sick." Jack shook his head. "I always thought you fellas were supposed to cure sickness, not cause it."

"You got me there. But you know what he meant, don't you?"

Jack nodded. "Just havin' a little fun with you, Doc." For a fleeting second, a cloud seemed to pass over his face, but an exuberant smile quickly replaced it. "I know nothing about chemotherapy except it won't be any picnic. What do you want to know next?"

I hesitated, then plunged ahead. "Did he discuss the prognosis with you?"

Jack briefly frowned. "You mean whether the treatments will work?"

"Yes. What's your understanding of the outlook? Did he discuss that with you?"

He sighed and turned his head to study the leaves of an oak tree gently fluttering in the morning breeze outside his window. After several seconds, he looked me in the face. "Yeah, he's a real cheerful fellow. Told me I'll die soon and to get my house in order, or something like that."

A pregnant silence followed for a long minute as Jack sat staring at the floor while I searched for comforting words to say. I shook my head sadly. "Well, Jack, I don't know quite what to say."

He looked up at me, his brief despair replaced with the glow of a beautiful smile. "You don't need to say anything, Doc. I know you're concerned about me and my mental health. Everyone thinks I've lost my mind because I'm not scared to death, but I remember you told me once that I needed to keep a positive attitude to recover from illness or any major reverse in life. I'm not at all in denial about my situation, but a pity party won't help me now. Understood?"

"Sure. You're right. I just wanted to be sure you understood the seriousness of stomach cancer."

"Doc, you know that I'm a Christian."

"Right. I'm thrilled about that."

"The way I look at it this is an opportunity to trust God. He's my heavenly Father and has my ultimate good in His mind and in His plans. Isn't that what you believe too?"

"I certainly do."

"Well, then my attitude is no mystery. If I live, I get to care for my family and see my kids married before I die." Although he still smiled, a single tear trickled down his right cheek as he sought for words to express his feelings. "If I die, I get to be with my earthly father and mother and my heavenly Father as we wait on the rest of the family to join us in God's tomorrow. That's a wonderful outcome, don't you think?"

"Yes, it is. You have a wonderful outlook, and I believe it will contribute to your recovery."

Jack nodded vigorously. "I worry about my son, William. He's never confessed a belief in Christ. So I spend my days in prayer for him especially. My Janie and our Lynn are strong Christians. I'm not so worried about them, although I don't want to leave them before I have to. My prayer is that William will come to know the Lord. And you know what else?"

I could only smile and shake my head as I awaited the answer.

"The Lord has promised me I will live to see William become a Christian and also to see Lynn happily married." At my surprised look, he laughed aloud. "I know. I know. Lynn doesn't even have a boyfriend right now. But I know that God answers prayer. Do you have time for me to tell you another quick story?"

"Sure thing. Go right ahead."

"When I was only ten years old, I loved walking in the woods with

Trapper, my old hound dog. One winter morning, I had the day off from school. I think it was on Christmas vacation. Anyway, we were far over in the deep woods behind the old home place when a tremendous snowstorm blew up. I remember thinking it was a grand adventure at first, but the snow fell so thick and fast that soon we couldn't see where we were going. To make matters worse, Trapper ran off to chase a rabbit, and I got good and lost.

"I wandered around in the blinding storm as snow fell heavily, bullets of sleet stung my face, and the winds picked up creating a blizzard that lasted a few hours. Unable to hear Trapper barking after a little while, I must have wandered in circles until I finally sat down huddled against a tree trunk, shivering with fear and the unrelenting cold. Although only a boy, I thought my hour had come. I tell you, I prayed like my life depended on it, and I'm sure it did. There in the storm, I first became acquainted with the Good Shepherd. I knew enough from Sunday school to confess my sins and ask for mercy."

Jack stared out the window again, pausing as he relived that life-changing experience in the dangerous storm so many years ago. He turned back to face me and continued his story. "Doc, I knew from that day on that my sins were forgiven. A peace I still cannot describe came over me that day. I've never gotten over that wonderful experience. Even during my Army days in the vicious fighting in the jungles of Viet Nam, I felt no debilitating fear. God's presence with me was too real for that. I was a sergeant leading a combat squad of men on my last tour of duty, and He was my constant companion in that time of extreme danger."

Tears moistened my eyes as a lump formed in my throat. I nodded and swallowed, unable to speak.

"You understand, Doc, that as an inexperienced boy, I faced what I believed was certain death that day in the deep woods. It turned out that I had wandered about two miles from home and was indeed in danger of dying from exposure right then and there. For about the seventh or eighth time I prayed that God would receive me into his home when I died. About then, I heard the deep baying of Trapper and the faint sound of my father shouting in the distance, calling my name. Well, it wasn't long before Trapper's cold nose nuzzled my face and his tongue kissed away my frozen tears while I hugged him tight. My father soon appeared out of the snowstorm and gathered me up in his firm arms to carry me home." His voice broke.

When he could go on, he said, "So, you see. I've already had a profound brush with death as a child. I was lost for about seven hours in dangerous frigid winter weather, inadequately dressed to face the intense freezing, blowing sleet, and snow. Since then, I've not been afraid to die. I know my heavenly Father will come to carry me home when He's ready for me, just like my dad did on that long-ago day. But now is not the time. I had a vivid dream last night about heaven. I saw Mom and Dad sitting at the feet of Jesus. They told me they weren't ready for me yet. I have family and friends to win for the Lord before I make my last journey. They told me it would be a matter of years. So you see, I don't worry."

I took a deep breath. "That's quite a story. You are a man of great faith."

I finished my examination of his heart and lungs. Dr. Hendrick had already changed his dressing and checked his abdominal wounds, so I didn't have to worry about that. As I prepared to leave, Jack reached out to shake my hand.

I gripped his hand in both of mine. "Thanks for telling me that inspiring story. I came to encourage you. Instead, you encouraged me."

Jack smiled again. "I appreciate you, Doctor. Thanks for listening and for not blowing me off as some kind of crackpot. I achieve my daily peace and balance by concentrating on prayer, controlling the thoughts that enter my mind, and reading God's Word, especially all the promises in the Bible. Don't you worry about me. I'll be fine."

Before leaving, I said, "I'm sure you will be, my friend."

CHAPTER 8—CRISIS

The next week on Friday, I finished early in the office for a change. Glancing at my watch and noting the time, 3:55 p.m., I couldn't believe it. No more patients to see until Saturday morning clinic hours. I heaved a sigh of relief and had a sudden inspiration.

Hurrying to the waiting room, I encountered Donna straightening up while Christine locked the front door. "Are we really finished early?"

Christine turned around and smiled. "We sure are."

"How did we accomplish that? We haven't finished this early in at least a year. In fact, I can't remember the last time we even came close, except during the blizzard last winter when the storm kept most people home."

Donna blushed as she turned in my direction. "We sort of arranged it. I hope you don't mind too much."

I assumed a stern countenance. "How did you 'sort of' arrange this early quitting time?"

She shrugged and looked at Christine. "It was her idea."

I folded my arms while continuing to scowl at the two of them.

Christine flushed, for once momentarily at a loss for words. At last, she found her voice. "It was my idea, but Donna was all for it. We kind a thought you needed a rest." She studied her feet for a few moments during the ensuing silence, then looked back up at me.

I struggled to continue my look of disapproval. "I'm sure there's more to it than that. I've never seen two more guilty-looking people in my life."

Christine took a deep breath. "I thought we needed a rest too," she said softly.

Donna noticed my lack of seriousness first and broke into a smile. "She has a date in a couple of hours."

I turned my stare on Christine. "Well?"

Beet red now, Christine couldn't say a word and looked pleadingly toward Donna for help.

Unable to continue the charade, my shoulders shook as I enjoyed a hearty laugh. "I'm sorry, Christine, but this is the first time I've seen you tongue-tied. Who's the lucky guy?"

Christine fanned herself with a magazine. "Doc, you scared me to death. I thought I was being fired."

I sat down across the room, waiting for them to regain enough composure to give me the details. Sensing the continued embarrassment, I let them in on my plans. "Actually, I agree with you. We all need a rest this evening. Thanks for arranging it. I plan to call Janet to see if she can get the kids ready for dining out this evening. She needs a break too." I paused briefly before continuing, "I still don't know who the lucky guy is."

Christine sighed in relief. "I'm sure glad you aren't mad at us. And actually, there are two guys."

Donna was blushing again, so I had a little more fun. "You mean you're going out with two guys at once? I would never have thought it of you."

Christine huffed. "Now, Doc. You know me better than that. Donna and I are going on a double date tonight."

"Really?"

"Really. You know that good-looking Marty Blackwell?"

I nodded. "Our illustrious deputy town marshal."

"Well, his cousin from Glen Falls is just as handsome. Marty asked me out, and his cousin Jeff is coming along and asked Donna to be his date tonight."

I smiled and stood up. "That's wonderful, ladies. If Jeff is as charming as his cousin, it sounds like this evening is a real winner for both of you."

Donna got up. "It was all Christine and Marty's doing, but I have to admit that I'm looking forward to this evening. Christine has already checked out Jeff thoroughly and finds that he is a gentleman and available. Wish us luck, Doc."

"Good luck to both of you. Now to surprise my wife and arrange for our family date."

∼

THREE HOURS LATER, I helped my wife seat our three children at our favorite Bob Evans restaurant in Indianapolis. We had enjoyed the opportunity to talk and relax during the fifty-minute drive to the city, and we both loved the barbecue rib dinners. There were plenty of items on the children's menu for our three little ones to choose from. Five-year-old Cindy and three-year-old twins Diane and David were engrossed in coloring pictures while we waited for the meal after placing our order. It was good to enjoy an evening out with the family.

The food was delicious, the atmosphere relaxing, and the children well behaved except for a minor incident involving which twin got to use the green crayon first. Our waitress enjoyed our children and supplied them with extra crayons and pictures to draw on when she noticed the problem of inadequate green crayons. After dining, Janet and I sat sipping iced tea with a lemon added for flavoring, discussing the day's events, and sharing the moment with pleasure.

Janet set her drink down. "So tell me about the girls' dates. It sounds so exciting."

"You know Marty Blackwell, our Glen Oaks deputy marshal?"

"Isn't he the one who had Guillain-Barre syndrome?"

"That's right. He made a complete recovery. Still, I thought he was making a lot of unnecessary appointments to be seen the last few weeks, but he must have been working up his nerve to ask Christine out. The office visits must have been an excuse to see her. He's as healthy as a young bull and just as strong. No sign of weakness or paralysis in him. Christine's had a crush on him since the first time he came to the office."

"I hope he's a suitable match for her. She's such a sweet girl."

"A sweet girl and a character!"

"Anyway, I hope she and Donna are having an enjoyable time. They both deserve the very best of companions. Everyone seems to love them."

"I'll admit, they really help my office practice shine," I said. "I just hope they don't both get married right away and quit on me."

Janet raised her eyebrows. "Now, Carl. You want what's best for them, don't you?"

I smiled and reached across the table to squeeze her hand. "You know I do. I just don't want to lose them yet. They'll be hard to replace."

"I'm sure they will be, but I don't think they'll be leaving you for a while. Most young couples need extra money, especially with the current inflation rate and the cost of living going up all the time. Besides, they aren't even engaged yet. This is just the first date. Give them some time. We don't even know how it will turn out, but you're right, they contribute so much to your office."

I squeezed Janet's hand again as I lost myself in the depths of her smile and sparkling eyes. She had a way of making me forget my problems.

That was when my beeper squawked its annoying alarm, spoiling a perfect evening with my family. Sighing, I reached down to my belt clip and turned it off.

The waitress approached, bringing the children's ice cream desserts, as I pushed back my chair to find a pay phone.

Nodding at me, Janet gave me her usual smile of encouragement. "I'll have the kids hurry in case you need to leave for an emergency."

The waitress advised me of pay phones in the hallway beside the restrooms, so I hurried and fortunately found one of three unoccupied at the moment.

The familiar voice of Rose Adams, hospital operator, answered in her usual soothing voice. "Glen Falls Hospital, how may I direct your call?"

"Hello, Rose. This is Dr. Matlock. You just paged me."

"Oh, yes. Vivian Crawford on surgery needs to speak with you about one of your patients. Just a moment while I ring you through."

As I waited for surgery to answer, my heart pounded in my throat. Vivian, a surgery charge nurse on the evening shift, was not one likely to call for minor problems. Jack O'Conner was my only patient still on the surgery floor, and he was due for release tomorrow. My concern for him resurfaced with a vengeance.

The line clicked as she connected with the surgery floor, and Rose announced my call. "I have Dr. Matlock on the line. Go ahead, please."

"Dr. Matlock, this is Vivian. I need you to check on Jack O'Conner. He's not doing well this evening. For the last hour he has been complaining of shortness of breath and heart palpitations. His BP is 140/100 with a pulse of 115, somewhat irregular. Respirations are 28 with an oral temp of 100.5. His color is poor. I started him on oxygen at 2 liters per minute by nasal canula and it seems to help a little. He's alert and cooperative but appears to be acutely ill. What orders do you have for me?"

"Unfortunately, I'm in Indianapolis dining out with my family. We were just finishing, so I'll start back right away. Does he look like he might code?"

"I don't think so, but you never know. Would you like me to get some lab work started on him?"

"Sure thing. Have radiology do a stat bedside upright chest film if he can sit up. Also, get stat arterial blood gases, CBC, chem 23 profile, blood cultures times two, and a UA. Does he have any orthostasis when he is upright in bed?"

"I knew you would ask, and one of the medical assistants is trying to get a BP and pulse with him sitting upright in bed as we speak. If you can hold on for a minute, I should have the answer for you shortly. I'll put you on hold if you don't mind."

"That's fine. I'll wait." I reviewed the multiple problems that could go wrong post-operatively from any major surgery while I waited for Vivian to come back on the line: myocardial infarction, pneumonia, cardiac arrhythmias, sepsis, delayed wound infection, abdominal abscess, organ perforation, pulmonary embolism, and the list went on.

Vivian's calm voice came back over the phone. "Doctor, his vital signs are about the same when he's positioned upright in bed. No evidence of orthostasis. He is also getting more relief with the oxygen. May I increase the oxygen if he seems to need it?"

"Yes, you can go up to 4 liters per minute as needed. Also, please get a stat EKG and an abdominal x-ray, a KUB. I'll gather my family up and try to be there in about an hour. I'll drop my family off at home unless you need me sooner. If you do, just have Rose page me rapidly twice in a row so I'll know to come straight to the hospital."

"Will do. Drive carefully. I can always call Dr. Neal in the ER for help if he deteriorates. He always helps when we need him."

That made me feel better. "Yes, call Dr. Neal if you need to. He's very competent."

I returned to our table to find that Janet already had the kids cleaned up from their ice cream spills and ready to go. Such was the life of a dedicated woman who marries a country doctor.

CHAPTER 9—BRUSH WITH DEATH

*A*fter an anxious drive, I arrived at Glen Falls Hospital at about 10:45 p.m. My beeper sounded no further alarms, so I had dropped my family off at home. Still, I remained apprehensive about Jack O'Conner as I rushed to the elevator for the third-floor surgical ward.

Vivian Crawford met me at the nurses' station and handed me Jack's chart with the EKG and vital signs attached to a separate clipboard. "You got here faster than I thought you would, but I'm glad to see you. Mr. O'Conner's pulse is much more irregular now. I took the liberty to ask for a repeat EKG. I hope you approve. The first one looked to me like sinus rhythm with tachycardia, but I don't think he's in sinus rhythm at this time."

"It's good that you ordered the test. Initiative in an emergency is praiseworthy, and I'm glad you got on it right away. The cardiology tech wheeled the electrocardiographic machine down the hallway as I got off the elevator. I'll write the order to cover you for the repeat EKG as I review the chart."

"Thanks, Doctor. I knew you wouldn't mind, but I wouldn't dare do that for some of your colleagues. And I'm sure you know who I mean."

I had to chuckle. "Yes, I understand, but I appreciate your aggressiveness in caring for a sick patient."

Leslie Farley, our efficient cardiology tech, interrupted our conversation to hand me the repeat EKG. "You'd better look at this right away. He's definitely had a change from the tracing I did earlier."

I quickly unrolled the twelve-lead standard EKG recording, as she hadn't had time to mount it in the chart. "He's in atrial fibrillation with a rapid ventricular response rate with non-specific ST-T wave changes, especially across the precordial leads. You're right. This is worrisome."

Vivian unrolled the first EKG strip and laid it on the desk so I could review them side by side. "I'd better go check on Mr. O'Conner and relieve Ann. She's our night supervisor and got here early to make rounds before the eleven o'clock change of shift. She relieved me at the bedside so I could answer the call lights of two other patients—nothing serious, but urgent needs."

"Ann Kilgore is working tonight?"

"Yes, she's always good to jump in and help with the floor work."

"That's good. She knows the family. They live on the same street in Glen Oaks. Jack will be glad she's on duty, I'm sure. Has the family been informed of his condition?"

"I called them about twenty minutes ago. They'll probably be here soon."

I glanced up at Vivian. "You were sure right about a change. The original EKG only showed sinus tachycardia but was normal otherwise. This repeat EKG with the new onset atrial fibrillation may represent a heart attack or a pulmonary embolism, among other possibilities." Vivian accompanied me as I hurried to Jack's room. "We need to transfer Jack to ICU. I hope there are open beds available. Have you checked the census with Ann yet?"

"Not yet, but I'm sure ICU isn't full tonight."

Ann had Jack sitting up at a sixty-degree angle so he could breathe better. One glance told me he was in trouble. Sweat dripped from his forehead as he struggled to get a deep breath. His lips and nail beds were cyanotic, and his speech limited to brief clipped words.

Ann had just restarted his IV with normal saline and was taping it in place when she looked up. "Good to see you, Doc. I can't make Jack behave tonight. He seems intent on spoiling my shift before it's even started."

Jack attempted a wan smile but gave up. Shaking his head, he nodded toward Ann and mouthed the word, "Character."

"Please help me lean him forward so I can listen to his back," I said.

Vivian on one side and Ann on the other supported him as I took a quick listen with my stethoscope. I nodded, and they eased him back to a semi-recumbent position supported by the elevated head of the bed so I could finish listening to his heart and lungs anteriorly. Finally, I palpated his abdomen and checked his lower extremities, noting mild swelling and exquisite tenderness to manual compression of his left calf.

"I believe there is a blood clot in the left leg, Jack. I suspect some of it has broken loose and traveled to your lungs."

Jack merely nodded.

Vivian patted his shoulder while Ann wiped sweat from his forehead and damp hair. Ann spoke first. "ICU bed?"

"Right. We need to move you where we can monitor you tonight, Jack. These ladies will try spoiling you."

Ann pulled her notes from a side pocket in her uniform, studied them, then announced, "Gotcha a bed. I'll call some extra help to get you moved down one floor to the ICU, okay, Jack? It'll just be a couple of minutes."

Ann handed me her brief notes with his vital signs scribbled at the bottom of the pad: BP 90/60, pulse 125 and irregular, respirations 32 and labored. "May I turn his oxygen up?"

"Yes, and let's get respiratory therapy here to change him to a non-rebreather mask at 100% oxygen and give him an albuterol inhalation treatment stat prior to transfer. He has diminished breath sounds on the lower right with distant wheezing in the same area of the lungs."

Leslie hovered outside the doorway, listening to our conversation. "That would be me tonight. I'm doubling as cardiology and respiratory tech this weekend on evening shifts, and I thought you'd have more orders for me."

I smiled. "Jack, with such expert help, I don't know if these ladies need me here or not, but I'll stay a while until you're better. All right with you?"

Jack gave my hand a brief squeeze, then whispered, "Thanks. Glad you're all here."

〰

TWENTY MINUTES LATER, Jack was in the ICU and breathing a little better following the albuterol inhalation treatment given on the surgery floor. Follow-up examination revealed improved air exchange with less bronchospasm but with continued diminished breath sounds in the right lower lobe. He still sat tilted up at sixty degrees, but with improved color and minimal diaphoresis. I knew he was getting better when he glanced up at me, winked, and gave his usual smile. "Scared you, didn't I?"

I took a deep breath. "You sure did. Why did you want to do a thing like that?"

Peggy Wilson and Liz O'Conner, a cousin of Jack's, bustled about the bed arranging the IV pole, checking the monitor leads, and straightening out the bedsheets. "He's just ornery, always has been, always will be," Liz said. She patted his shoulder, grinning all the while. "Actually, Jack's my favorite cousin. I'll enjoy bossing him around for a while. He's always been a big tease. Never able to keep his mouth shut."

"You'd better watch yourself tonight," I told him. "These nurses will not tolerate any more of your shenanigans."

Peggy finished rechecking his vital signs. "BP 120/90, pulse 91. Would you like me to slow the IV down? He's had 1000 ml now."

"Yes, slow the infusion rate to 125 ml per hour and monitor I&O hourly. He doesn't have a Foley catheter in for hourly monitoring of his

59

output, but I believe he can cooperate well enough to empty his bladder frequently without one in place."

Jack nodded. "No catheters, please."

"You understand the need for an accurate I&O, don't you?"

"Right. You want to measure how much I take in and how much I put out, so you can tell if my kidneys are functioning okay. I'm no dummy, you know."

Peggy nodded. "He's getting better, all right. But he has to rest, and he's talking too much. Doc, please go write your orders while we finish settling him in bed." She winked at me, knowing I wouldn't take offense at her banter. She was also one of my patients who'd had her own brush with death in the past with a ruptured ectopic pregnancy and shock.

Just then, Sally Walker, our radiology tech, entered the ICU with Jack's portable chest film and mounted it on the x-ray view box. "Do you need any more films done?"

"Not tonight. This one is fine." I traced the vague opacity in the right lower lobe with my finger as I studied the chest film. "This may be an area of infarction or atelectasis. I'll want a repeat chest film in the morning to check this area again."

"I'll leave a note for day shift to get one first thing in the morning."

Ann came through the automatic doors just as Sally prepared to leave. "I've got Jack's family in the ICU waiting room outside whenever you're ready to see them."

"Give me a few minutes to finish his orders. Then I'll be right there."

"Okay. I'll wait with them. Janie is nearly frantic. I'll let her know that he's doing a lot better and appears to be stabilizing."

I finished studying Jack's stat labs, noting the pronounced hypoxemia and hyperventilation with a pO2 of 50 and pCO2 of 27 on the initial blood gases completed after my initial telephone orders from the restaurant. Finishing up, I ordered more coagulation studies for the morning to compare with his baseline levels and ordered the initiation of Heparin for anticoagulation therapy for presumed pulmonary embolus with a small pulmonary infarction.

On my way out, I stopped by Jack's bed. "How are you doing?"

"There's a little sharp pain in my right chest when I try to take a deep breath now. I also coughed up a little blood after they got me settled in bed."

"It's likely that you have a blood clot in your right lung. I'll let Dr. Hendrick know in the morning. One thing is for sure. You'll be spending more time with us in the hospital."

Jack was lying down at about fifteen degrees elevation, resting comfortably as I turned to go. "Wait up." He stretched out his right hand to clasp mine as I turned back around. "Thanks, Doc. Thanks a lot. Don't worry too much about me. It's still not my time to go. And send my family home to get some rest."

~

JANIE JUMPED up from the ICU waiting room couch as I approached. "Is Jack going to be okay? Is he dying?"

Ann rose from her chair and moved beside Janie and gave her a gentle hug. William, pacing like a caged tiger, wheeled about to face me while Lynn sat in a corner wiping her eyes with a handkerchief.

William glared at me. "Yeah, what's going on here? Did somebody do something wrong?"

Lynn cleared her throat. "Stop it, William. Nobody did anything wrong. I already told you that."

"Yeah, well, what do you know? You're not a doctor yet. Maybe you'll never be one."

"I'm smart enough to mind my manners and to wait for information before jumping to stupid conclusions."

Janie wrung her hands. "Children, please stop."

William backed off, muttering, as Lynn answered, "It's all right, Mother. He's just feeling guilty for the way he ignores Dad's counsel. Now he thinks he has to make up for it by his overly protective macho behavior."

61

It was time to intervene. "Actually, he's stable and improving. Let's all sit down so we can discuss what's happened and the course of action I've started for his treatment."

Ann helped Janie back to her seat and encouraged William to sit by his mother. "Would any of you like some coffee? I just made a fresh pot for the ICU staff. There's plenty for all."

Janie nodded. "Thanks. I could use a cup right now."

"William? Lynn? How about it?"

They both nodded, and Ann hastened to bring them refreshments.

I sat across from Janie and William while Lynn remained in the corner to my right. Folding my hands in my lap, I cleared my throat. "You all know that Jack was doing well until today. He is a stoical man and didn't tell anyone that his left leg was swelling and painful until after the crisis began."

William looked skeptical, but Lynn leaned forward attentively and put her hand over her mouth. "Oh, I bet he had a blood clot in his leg that became an embolus to his lungs!"

I nodded. "Exactly right. I'm convinced that's what happened."

William shook his head. "So, are you going to take the blood clot out?"

Lynn rolled her eyes and slouched back in her chair.

Janie blotted tears with a tissue as she slowly regained control of her emotions. "Now I want both of you quiet while the doctor helps me understand your father's condition. Lynn, I appreciate your quick grasp of the situation, but I'm still mystified. William, I know you love your father, although you've had several disagreements with him recently. You may be eighteen, but I can still make you sorry. Understand?"

Lynn nodded. "Sorry, Mother."

William shrugged, still scowling. "Okay, Mom."

Ann returned just then with a tray full of steaming-hot coffee mugs, one for each of us. I took a sip from mine and set it on the table beside my chair. "Jack is a determined man with a mind of his own. He's much better now and just informed me this is not his time to die. He understands this is a life-threatening condition, but he seems to have an assurance he will be fine." I grinned at Lynn. "In fact, he recently told me he will walk you down the aisle and give you away someday and live to attend your med school graduation."

Lynn blushed but looked pleased.

It was William's turn to roll his eyes, but he was careful to keep his mouth closed and his face turned away from his mother.

I let my last statement sink in for a moment before continuing, "Jack has several risk factors for a blood clot and subsequent pulmonary embolus. First, there is surgery as a risk factor. Blood coagulation is affected by surgical procedures. Also, cancer predisposes to clotting abnormalities. Finally, he has been mostly at bedrest and fairly inactive for once in his life. He's done his best to walk in the hallway, but it still happened despite his best effort at mobility."

Lynn nodded in understanding but looked perplexed. "What about his heart? Ann mentioned a rhythm problem."

"I believe the arrhythmia is secondary to the primary event, the embolism. A pulmonary embolus puts a temporary strain on the right heart, causing sudden engorgement because of back pressure from the clot lodging in the lungs. That life-threatening development can trigger atrial arrhythmias. He developed atrial fibrillation initially but is back in a sinus rhythm. Have you studied atrial fibrillation yet?"

"A little. I know it's a disorganized, frequently rapid arrhythmia. I didn't realize that an embolus could cause it, but I got your explanation okay. So does his repeat EKG look normal?"

Ann stood again. "The girls were just doing the EKG. I'll get it for you to review." Within moments, Ann returned with the EKG.

I spread it out so they could all see the tracing. "Notice how regular it is now."

William nodded. "Even I can see that."

Lynn smiled. "Daddy's heart is in sinus rhythm. I'm not sure, but I think the last EKG is normal."

"Lynn, you just passed EKG Reading 101. It's perfectly normal, an excellent sign."

Janie shook her head. "I don't understand everything you two are saying, but I believe it means he's getting better. Am I right?"

"Yes. I've started him on anticoagulation with IV Heparin. In the morning, I'll start low-dose oral Coumadin. That should prevent more clots from developing and the current thrombus from extending the damage. His body will have to eventually dissolve or otherwise deal with the clots that have already formed. We don't have a way of dissolving them at the present time. Maybe Lynn will someday have the advantage of a drug that will dissolve clots in her patients. Remember, he's not totally out of danger, but he's much, much better. So, who wants to come with me to visit with him?"

William spoke up first. "We're all ready to see Dad. And, Doc, I'm sorry for what I said. Guess I was a little excited."

"You're just stressed out," I said. "Now let's all go in, but only for a few minutes."

CHAPTER 10—THE STORM

$\mathcal{A}$ blinding flash of light accompanied by an ear-splitting thunderclap shattered the peace of the early morning darkness. Janet stumbled out of bed, grabbed her robe, and ran to check on the children. Awake now but feeling disoriented, I propped myself up on my elbow. "What was that?"

Lightning illuminated the darkness of our bedroom as thumber rumbled ominously, rattling the windowpanes. The weather radio popped on, sounding a piercing alarm as a monotone voice announced a severe storm warning. "This is NOAA Weather Station in Glen Falls, Indiana. The Indianapolis Airport radar system has detected a powerful line of storms moving through central and southern Indiana east of Indianapolis. This is a dangerous weather system with likely damaging winds, large hail, and possible tornado activity. The following counties are affected…"

Shaking my head to clear my thoughts, I glanced at the luminous dial of the bedside clock: 4:00 a.m. Had it only been four hours ago that I pillowed my head after checking on Jack O'Conner following the pulmonary embolism?

Flickering light from the storm lit up our bedroom as Janet returned with our twins each clinging to one of her hands. Cindy followed with her teddy bear tucked under her right arm and Janet's robe tightly clinched in her left hand.

The emergency warning sirens activated, wailing loudly from high atop the feed mill in downtown Glen Oaks just as the clock dial faded out and the weather radio lost about half of its volume as battery power took over.

The children whimpered.

Fully awake now, I fumbled in the darkness searching for my slippers and the flashlight at the head of the bed. "We just lost our electricity. Maybe we'd better go to the basement and take the weather radio along. It will be safer there until the worst of the storm passes over. The weather station will keep us posted about the storm and let us know when it's all clear to come back upstairs."

"I'm scared," Cindy said.

"Shush, children," Janet soothed them. "It's okay. Daddy will find a light, and Jesus is always with us. Remember your Sunday school lesson last week? Jesus stilled a storm on an enormous lake because the disciples were afraid. He cared for them, and He will care for us."

After I found and switched on the flashlight, its warm beam of light pushed back the frightening shadows and comforted the children. I quickly shined it about the room and located a second smaller flashlight, which I handed to Cindy. "Please shine the way for your mother and the twins to get to the basement. I'll be right down. I want to take a quick look out the windows and see if that first lightning bolt hit one of our trees. It struck close to our house for sure."

Making my way from room to room, trying to see the trees nearest the house, I gave up when a roaring deluge of rain and wind lashed our home, making it impossible to see anything outside with clarity. Things appeared to take a turn for the worse as large hail began drumming on the roof and sides of the house.

I joined Janet and the children in the safety of the basement, where she snuggled with all three in a comfortable over-sized brown rocking chair. The children quieted as she crooned familiar lullabies to them. A battery-operated lantern we used for night fishing on the nearby lake substituted for the flashlights, as we hoped to conserve their batteries for possible later use. Finding a chair nearby, I listened intently to the weather but with mixed reception from the basement. Lots of static and squealing interfered with normal programing.

Radio reception improved on NOAA as the storm abated at 4:35 a.m. Signaling my intention to Janet, I retrieved the larger flashlight and ascended to the main floor of our home to check things out.

The eerie whistling of the wind gave way to the gentle patter of rain hitting the house while water continued to gush down the drainpipes with a loud rushing, gurgling sound. Faint streaks of gray lightened the eastern sky with the hopeful promise of a peaceful dawn. The warning sirens downtown had ceased. Unfortunately, we still had no electricity. That would likely not be restored for hours, judging by the intensity of the recent storm.

Satisfied that the worst was over, I signaled that it appeared safe to return from sheltering in the basement. As three relieved and energetic children spilled into the kitchen from the basement stairway, I had to smile. Janet followed close behind with the second flashlight and the lantern as three little voices now clamored for breakfast. Cindy took the lead as usual. "Mommy, we're hungry. Can we have some ham and eggs?"

"I'm afraid not. We don't have electricity to cook with until the power company turns the lights back on. Ours is an electric stove. It won't work until we get our power back."

Disappointment wreathed three little faces illuminated by light from the lantern now on the kitchen table.

Janet smiled and clapped her hands together. "But I have a splendid idea. How about peanut butter and jelly? Sound good?"

Instantly, sorrow turned to bliss as smiles replaced frowns and long faces. Joining in with the change of atmosphere, I offered support. "Sounds wonderful. I'll get the pitcher of milk from the refrigerator and pour our drinks to go along with the sandwiches. This has been an exciting adventure to begin Saturday morning."

～

DURING THE DRIVE back from morning rounds at the hospital, I watched the last of the black storm clouds scudding to the east as the sun broke through in dazzling brilliance and a striking rainbow arched over the interstate from horizon to horizon. Downed power lines, fallen trees, and ponding water on the road all added to the hazards of being out and about.

Shaking my head, I wondered what I would find at the office. Communication had been completely cut off after the violence of the morning storm. Downed telephone lines east of Glen Falls. A real mess for local authorities.

After I turned off the interstate, the last three or four miles back into town were the biggest challenge. Luckily, I had taken a different route to the hospital earlier and had only a few brief delays finding my way around downed trees across the roads. Some secondary roads were water covered and impassable according to the county sheriff I conversed with at the hospital.

Instead of the usual five-minute drive into Glen Oaks, frequent detours because of road outages delayed my arrival at the office by another twenty minutes. It was a relief to see two cars in the parking lot belonging to my staff, but the darkened appearance of the office itself was disconcerting.

After parking in my usual spot behind the office, I hurried to the back door wanting to survey the potential damage inside. The lights most definitely should have been on indoors. Downed tree limbs and leaves ripped from once-living trees covered the far side of the back parking lot. Hopefully the front windows were still intact.

As I placed my key in the lock, the door jerked open to reveal Christine breathing a sigh of relief. "Thank goodness you're safe. We heard some homes in your part of town sustained a lot of wind damage. There's already a rumor that the storm killed someone. Apparently, a tornado ripped through town along with the storm. Did you see any collapsed houses? Is your family okay? Is your house still standing? I've been really worried."

Christine was just being Christine as usual, and I smiled. "Whoa, hold on a second. I appreciate your concern, but other than losing our electricity, we're okay. There is some wind debris in the yard to clean up later today, but that's a minor problem."

Donna entered the room from the front hallway door. She rolled her eyes and shook her head. "I'm glad you're here too. Christine has been regaling me with horror stories about injuries you've probably sustained. We couldn't get you on the phone, but with the lines down, that's not too surprising. If I die with a heart attack, it's all her fault."

Christine whirled around, scowling at Donna. "You had your nightmare scenarios of destruction, death, and decapitation too. You're no better than me. Besides, it just shows how much we care about Doc and his family. So, there!"

Time to intervene. "Ladies, I appreciate your concern, but we're fine. Is there any damage to the front office or waiting room?"

Donna shook her head. "None that I could see, but the front lot is a mess with leaves, tree limbs, and even trash cans blowing around in the wind."

"If the patients can find a place to park, I'll worry about that later."

Christine pulled out a chair and sat down at our break table. "I don't know how I'll get through the morning. Can't even make coffee with the electricity off. My nerves are frazzled."

Donna crossed the room to sit beside her. "How are we going to see patients in the dark? Your office has a window with some light from outside, but the other exam rooms have no outside source of light at all."

I took a seat across from them. "What kind of schedule do we have this morning?"

Christine spread her hands wide apart. "A full schedule. The interesting part is whether anyone will show up."

"Let's think about it for a minute. Still no phone service?"

Christine frowned and shook her head. "None. Next question."

I had to chuckle. "Obviously, no light source except for flashlights."

Christine crossed her arms over her chest. "None."

Donna nudged her with an elbow. "You're good with that word. Do you know any others?"

Christine started to respond, but I held up my hands. "Ladies, truce. You can argue after hours all you want."

Christine stuck her tongue out at Donna. "I can hardly wait!"

Donna looked annoyed for a moment, but her sunny disposition could not be suppressed for long. She hugged Christine and beamed a smile in her direction. "Oh, come on. You know I'm just kidding. Still friends?"

Christine's phony façade dissolved as she laughed. "Sure. Still friends."

"Now that we have that solved, I suggest that Christine greet the patients as usual out front, explain the situation, and seat them in the waiting room. Donna can bring one at a time back here to the break room table where we have enough light from the picture window to work. Hopefully, no one needs an abdominal exam today. I think we can get by. It'll be slower, but we only have a half day to work."

"Doc, now that we have that settled, I want to know how Jack is this morning. I heard a rumor that he had an awful night."

Leave it to Christine to catch the early gossip. "What did you hear?"

"Well, I stopped by the drug store to see if they had anything for breakfast, what with the electricity out. All they had was cream-filled donuts and milk." She smiled. "Boy, were they good. I brought some extra if either of you are hungry."

"That doesn't tell me what you heard."

"Please, Doc. Don't spoil a magnificent story. I had to tell about the donuts. I heard he had to be moved to ICU because of some kind of clot.

Of course, I put little stock in it. You told us yesterday that he was doing very well."

I shook my head. Small town. No secrets. None. "I don't know how stories get around so fast in this town."

Donna nodded knowingly. "Constance Thorndike, no doubt. Our favorite histrionic, hysterical hypochondriac. I saw her leave the drug store as I drove into town."

Christine agreed, "Well, yes. She's some kind of third or fourth cousin of Jack's, two or three times removed supposedly. Being a hypochondriac doesn't make her news about someone else false."

"No, it doesn't. As a matter of fact, she's right. She lives across the street from the O'Conner family. She probably noticed them leaving late for the hospital last night. That alone would be enough to keep her up half the night waiting for any news. Unfortunately, Jack had a pulmonary embolus. I had to move him to ICU. Things looked serious for a while, but he improved and is much better this morning. If he's stable over the weekend, I plan to move him to a medical floor on Monday."

The bell over the front door jangled as the first patient entered out front. Christine jumped up to hurry to her desk.

"Just a minute. You don't get off that easy. How did your dates go last night?"

Christine whirled around, flushing a deep red. "You told him."

Donna spread her hands. "How could I have told him? You were here the whole time we talked."

"Told me what?"

Donna laughed. "The park was nice and cozy. The bench beside the pond was so romantic, and someone got a kiss."

Christine shook her fist at Donna. "Just you wait. I'll get even. You're just jealous that you didn't get kissed."

"His cousin is a perfect gentleman, and it was just our first date. I hardly know him, but we have another date next week."

Christine charged across the room, still beet red and muttering to herself.

Donna looked at me. "She's hopeless, but I think the world of her anyway. She's an exceptional friend. And we both will want more information about Jack after we close the office today."

CHAPTER 11—SADNESS AND CONFUSION

The morning passed quickly after we instituted our plan for working during the power outage. The combined break/medicine/lab room functioned adequately for patient visits as most of the scheduled appointments were for minor problems. All but one patient made it to the office following the storm. Still, we had no telephone service to contact anyone prior to 11:45. Outside, the temperature climbed rapidly along with the humidity. I mopped sweat from my forehead while waiting for Donna to bring in the last patient.

Donna brought in Emma Donaldson, escorted by her fifty-five-year-old son, Harvey, as I finished my visit notes on the previous patient. He smiled and extended his hand as I stood to greet them. "Good morning, Doctor. Mom wanted to see you today."

Harvey took a seat across from me at the end of the table next to the laboratory area while Donna seated Emma beside the table facing me. Emma placed her large purse on the table and sat up straight, hands folded tightly in her lap to control the tremor in her hands. She stared out the window behind me, watching the neighbor's horses in the pasture behind the office.

Emma sat silently while Donna bent beside her, checking vital signs.

"Your blood pressure is normal today, Emma. 125/70. Pulse 72 and regular." Donna glanced at me. "Do you want her temperature checked too?"

"What are you here to see me for today, Emma?" I asked.

Emma remained silent, fascinated with the horses outdoors.

"Is she sick today, Harvey?"

"No, she's looking for Dad and wanted to see you." Harvey raised his eyebrows and shrugged helplessly.

Emma could be difficult. "I think we'll skip the temperature for now. Let me check her over first."

Donna nodded and walked to the sink across the room to scrub her hands.

At that moment, the lights flickered on and the air conditioner hummed in the background, a most welcome sound.

Emma blinked her eyes and looked at her son. "What was that?"

Harvey smiled and patted her hand. "It's okay, Mom. The electricity just came back on. That's progress. The boys are working overtime on the power lines today."

I nodded. "The air conditioner is a relief. It must be boiling outside."

"It sure is. Mom doesn't do too well in air conditioning though. She prefers the temperature in the eighties. About runs sis and me out of the house. She keeps closing the windows to shut out any slight breeze. Sometimes it's hard to take, but we do our best to put up with it."

Emma became intense as she turned to focus out the window. "Could I borrow one of your horses?"

"I'm sorry. Those aren't my horses. They belong to our neighbor. You know Mark Applegate and his family, don't you?"

"Why are the horses here? Are they sick? Do you have to doctor them too?"

Harvey leaned over and gave her a quick hug. "Doc's not a veterinarian, Mom. Don't you remember Mark? Dad always liked him and his family. Those horses belong to him."

"Oh yes. Now I remember. Maybe he has seen Fred. We'll go there next. Thanks for your help, Doctor. You always know what to do." She started to stand until Harvey placed a restraining hand on her right shoulder.

He sighed and shook his head. "Don't you remember? Dad's been gone for twenty years. He died at sixty with a heart attack."

Emma appeared stunned. "I didn't know he was sick. We better go to the hospital if he's had a heart attack."

Harvey rested his elbows on the table and buried his head in his hands. "What can we do for her?" he asked me. "This goes on all day and sometimes half the night."

Not knowing what else to say, I looked at Emma. "Let me check your heart and lungs. I need to make sure you're okay."

"Whatever you say, Doctor, but please hurry. We need to go see Dad. Did you hear that he's had a heart attack? Have they called you to take care of him?"

For an eighty-year-old patient, her exam turned out to be normal, as was usual for her. Emma had experienced few sick days during her life, but the last five years had been difficult for the family as they watched her memory slip away. She often forgot about personal hygiene, self-care, and nutrition. She left burners lit on the stove and water running in the sink, and she had to be reminded to eat the meals her family set before her. Staying alone was no longer possible, not even for an hour. (It would be another sixteen years before the first medication for Alzheimer's disease hit the market. We had no idea it would take so long.)

Donna stood by, waiting for instruction as I completed the examination.

"Let's see if she can get a urine specimen for us," I said. "The light in the bathroom is on now, but you'd better stay with her to assist. One more thing, check her temperature. I don't want to miss an occult infection."

Donna nodded, smiled, and gently took Emma's hand. "Come on, Emma. Doc wants a urine test done."

Emma smiled up at her. "Is that a hard test? Do I need to study?"

Donna led her from the room. "It's easy. I'll tell you what to do. Okay?"

"As long as you're with me, honey, I'm sure it'll be okay. I have always liked you."

As their voices faded down the long hallway outside the lab door, Harvey straightened up in his chair. A solitary tear trickled down his right cheek. "It's hard, Doc. Seeing her that way breaks my heart. You know what I mean?"

"I'm so sorry. I only have a vague idea what you're going through. I admire you and Beverly for taking such excellent care of your mother. It is hard."

"Neither one of us is getting any younger. I'm not sure how long we'll be able to keep this up. Beverly is lucky to have an understanding family. She's with Mom more than she's at her own home. Lucky for sis, her oldest daughter is still at home and does most of the cooking and chores for the family. Beverly's husband is a kind, generous man, rarely complaining about the situation."

"It hurts to admit it, but unless your mother has an infection I can treat, there's little I have to offer."

Harvey stared at the floor. "I know. We're not blaming you. Her father, we called him Grandpop, had the same problem before he died. I didn't think we'd have to face this again after he died. Life sure is an uncertain proposition."

"There may come a time when you decide on nursing home care for your mother. You probably can't care for her at home indefinitely. If that time comes, I'll be happy to help you with admitting her and caring for her in that setting. A sad fact of life is that the caretakers of a patient this impaired have a much greater chance of experiencing a major illness because of the stressful lifestyle."

Harvey nodded. "I don't doubt that at all. I'll talk it over with my sister again. Mom's incontinent half the time now. I know we're both exhausted. Beverly is fifty, and I'm no spring chicken." He managed a brief smile that soon faded. "It's so sad to see a deteriorating mind trapped in a healthy body. I'm glad now that Dad didn't live to see her like this. It would've broken his heart."

"I know."

We sat in silence for a few minutes until Donna returned with Emma holding onto her arm. "Success! We got the urine, but it looks clear. Her temperature is normal. I'll have the dipstick results for you in a minute."

Emma smoothed her dress as she sat down. "She's a sweet girl. I hope she finds out what's wrong so she can get well."

Exasperated, Harvey shook his head and stood up. "Come on, Mom. Let's go to the waiting room while they run the tests."

"Sure, son. I want to know how she is before we leave. Where are we going next? I forgot already."

Harvey let out a long breath as he took her by the arm. "Come with me. We'll talk about it later. Thanks, Doc. I want to settle her bill while we're waiting. Besides, Christine always cheers me up. I could use her smiles and cheerful chatter today."

Donna looked my way as she finished writing the results in her chart. "Sorry. It's all normal. I hoped to find something you could treat. I really feel for the family. Poor Emma. She doesn't even realize what's going on."

"True, but it's a blessing that she doesn't know how far she has progressed with dementia already. I wish a cure could be found for Alzheimer's disease soon. Someday, there will be something we can offer besides condolences."

Within a short time, the ladies had the office cleaned up to prepare for Monday and I had put the finishing touches on the last charts. Christine poked her head in the lab door. "Doc, are you ready to tell us all about Jack O'Conner?"

"Sure, come on in. But I warn you, you must tell me all about your dates. Deal?"

77

She flushed again. "You drive a hard bargain, but okay. Deal! I won't rest all weekend until I know all the details about Jack."

I pushed back from the table, laughing. "You're too much. My wife enjoys the tales I bring home."

"That's okay, Doc. Janet's sweet. She won't repeat them."

CHAPTER 12—HOMEWARD BOUND

*J*ack sat on the side of the bed, fully dressed, tennis shoes on with laces tied, and the IV out of his arm. When I entered the room smiling, he looked up frowning. "It's about time you got here. I'm ready to get out of this place. Janie and Lynn are on the way to pick me up."

Eleven days had passed since his brush with death, and he looked great.

"It's only eight o'clock," I said. "Give me a break."

"I expected you at seven. What gives?"

As I took a seat, I winked at him. "Saved the best till last."

"Flattery won't help you. I was ready to leave two hours ago."

I patted his knee and started leafing through his chart. "I'll try to have your discharge completed by the time your family arrives."

Jack chuckled. "Had you going, didn't I?"

"You're not mad at me?"

"Nah. You should know better than that. Just having a little fun at your expense." He cleared his throat. "Seriously, I'm more than ready to get out of here. This place is wonderful when you need it, but it has a way of growing on you, and not in a pleasant way. I'm a patient man, but

79

if one more nurse comes to take my temperature, I'll have a hard time being civil."

"Sure you will." I grinned back. Jack loved drama, and he was still putting on an act. "We need to review some precautions and safety information. First, no aspirin, ibuprofen, or similar drugs. A lot of medications don't mix with Coumadin, and those are just two of them. Don't take over-the-counter medicine until you check with the office. If we don't have the answers, Barry House, our local pharmacist, can help us find them.

"Regarding trauma, you must be extra careful since you're on Coumadin to prevent another blood clot or abnormal blood loss. If you sustain an injury with bleeding, apply pressure and call me if it isn't controlled in five minutes. And please call immediately for any serious injuries. Major bruising can be a sign of serious internal bleeding. Also, if you notice any black tarry bowel movements, that could be caused by internal bleeding, and you must call at once.

"Finally, I want to see you in the office in two days to check on your progress. While you're there, Donna will draw your blood for a protime test to send to the hospital lab. Our goal is to keep your protime between one and a half and two times normal. With that information, the office can adjust your Coumadin dosage and decide when to test it next. Understood?"

"Sure, Doc. I'll be a pin cushion for several weeks until I can get off this medication. Right?"

"We prefer not to think of it in that way. It's for your own good."

Jack guffawed and slapped his knee. "That's what you always say before you come at me with needles and other diabolical painful procedures."

Shaking my head and smiling, I remained silent while he regained control of his emotions and did his best to maintain a brave front. He needed to let off steam.

Jack appeared thoughtful, even worried, after his joke. "Seriously, Doc. I remember what I told you about surviving this cancer, but sometimes late at night I get frightened and have trouble with my faith. Mostly, I'm concerned about my family. I'm the breadwinner in our house, and that's scary with cancer hanging over my head. What do you really think? Am I being too optimistic about my chances of survival?"

Not a question I relished answering. I took a deep breath, trying to think of an appropriate but reassuring response. "I can't say for sure. Only God knows the number of our days, both yours and mine. I once heard a wise minister say that we are immortal until God is finished with us here on earth. I only know that a positive attitude is necessary to battle any serious illness. Depression, defeatism, and doubt are all potential killers. I've seen some people give up and die long before their prognosis suggested it would happen. I've seen others who refused to accept an arbitrarily assigned date with death and lived life to the full for several years beyond any reasonable expectation by the experts."

"Makes sense." He leaned forward and clasped his hands together. "I promise you I'll be upbeat. I'm a fighter from way back. You should know that by now. Please don't misunderstand, I'm not afraid of dying. I'm just concerned about my family. I promised Janie that she wouldn't have to work outside the home when we were first married. I didn't want babysitters or daycare workers raising our kids. I know some women have to work, but I didn't want that for my family. I also want to see Lynn graduate from medical school, and I can't wait to walk her down the aisle and give her to her own prince charming. She deserves the best, Doc. She's never given us any serious problems."

"I'll do my best to help you accomplish your goals. You've already been an inspiration to me and the girls in the office."

Jack hesitated, choking up, suppressing a sob. "One more thing. I want to live long enough to see William settled spiritually in life. He's the one I'm most concerned about. William's another issue entirely. He's basically a good boy, but he's not a Christian and has a tendency to run around with the wrong crowd. I could die peacefully if I knew he had surrendered his life to the Lord. Please pray for him and ask your office staff to remember him in their prayers. I know they really care about people."

"I will give them your request. They'll be honored that you asked. Do you have any more questions before I sign your release papers?"

"No, that about does it for now. I'll think of a half dozen questions after you leave, but nothing comes to mind since you brought it up." He smiled as he warmly shook my hand with both of his. "Thanks, Doc. Thanks a lot. You and Doc Hendrick saved my life. However many days the Lord gives me, you both helped make it possible. I'm indebted."

"I'm thankful that you pulled through, my friend. We will beat this illness as a team. Call the office for any issues. Okay?"

"Will do. Better hurry with those orders. Lynn is standing behind you in the doorway, and I'm raring to go home."

CHAPTER 13—CHAOS IN THE OFFICE

a welcome cold front moved through Glen Oaks on Wednesday, bringing refreshing summer showers and dropping temperatures into the mid-seventies. At 9:00 a.m., the waiting room quickly filled as Christine registered patients at her office window and Donna hastened to prepare patients in the exam rooms. The ladies worked together with quiet efficiency, too busy to spend time in small talk for once.

Donna handed me the first charts at 9:10. "Three little sweethearts for you to see first. All here for well-child vaccinations."

I picked up the charts, glancing at the names. Mary Elizabeth, two-and-a-half-year-old daughter of Katy Richardson with meningomyelocele, father deceased, and child adopted by Michael Richardson. Ruth Marie, one-year-old with cerebral palsy, adopted by Michael and Katy Richardson. Finally, Robert Mills Richardson, eleven-month-old son of Michael and Katy, named in honor of Katy's deceased first husband, Robert Mills.[1]

Memories flooded my mind with equal emotions of both overwhelming sadness and joy as I recalled the years of tragedy and triumph experienced by these two young parents. With exemplary love and devotion to one another, they shared in raising Michael's three older children, Katy's handicapped daughter, an adopted daughter with cerebral palsy, and their own son, treating and loving all six alike. Not satisfied to care only for their six children, they had established the Robert Mills Memorial Fund to assist parents caring for handicapped children.

"A wonderful, closely knit family," Donna said. "I just love those children."

"You're right about that. Are the older children here today also?"

"No. Katy's parents are babysitting for them today. It's exciting to watch Clayton enjoying being a grandpa, even to children who aren't blood relatives. I didn't think he would be the type to enjoy this so much."

"As the old saying goes, wonders never cease. A stern middle-aged macho man turned into a push-over powder puff by the antics and love of little children. Amazing!"

"May I help with the exams? I've got the other exam rooms filled already, and those children are just too precious. I have to help hold the babies."

"Sure. Let's get started with the morning."

Donna laughed softly. "You'd better. The waiting room is packed, and we have a walk-in without an appointment—Johnny Morton."

"Can't you get him to come in later today?"

"Only if you don't mind letting him bleed all over town."

I groaned and paused before entering exam room 1. "Please tell me he's not been fishing."

Donna grinned wickedly. "Sorry, Doc. Johnny's been fishing all night."

"Another hook embedded in his hand?"

"Not just a hook, but a hook and a large lure with treble hooks, both in the same hand."

"If he's bleeding, does he need attention first?"

"No. Christine made him take his four-pound smallmouth bass back out to the car. He dripped blood on the waiting room carpet, showing off his catch. She'll bring him to the treatment area in the back to soak his hand in a basin after he stows the fish in his pickup. Johnny can wait a bit. He's been standing in the parking lot showing off his catch for at least five minutes. He won't bleed to death."

Reaching for the doorknob, I sighed. "I've got an ominous feeling about today. We're really off from the starting gate with a bang."

Michael stood to shake hands as I entered the room. "Something wrong, Doc?"

"Sorry. Not really. I didn't mean to sigh that loud. It has nothing to do with you."

He grinned. "I can guess. Johnny Morton nearly pulled my arm off getting me to come look at his catch in the truck. He grabbed me as soon as I opened the car door. I humored him briefly but excused myself to help Katy with the kids. Have you ever fished with him?"

"I'm afraid I haven't had the honor."

Michael snickered. "Do yourself a favor and don't. I went with him once last summer and he caught the seat of my pants with one of his vicious lures. Ruined a good pair of jeans cutting it out. He catches a lot of fish, but for the life of me, I don't know how. He spends a lot of time catching tree limbs, snags in the river, and his fishing buddies. It's a million laughs if you're short on entertainment."

"Thanks for the warning. I'll pass if he asks me. He's a likeable kid, but he sure lives on the edge."

Katy smiled pleasantly. "You should go fishing with him. Maybe you could tame him a little."

I shook my head. "No, thanks. Now, how are the little ones today?"

Donna brought in an extra chair and sat holding baby Robert, tickling his chin while he cooed at her. Katy helped me with the examinations while Michael held one little girl at a time in another chair. I examined them carefully. Both handicapped but fortunate to have such loving parents. Neither showed any fear or sign of alarm, as they were accustomed to seeing doctors, and me in particular.

Katy gave a running commentary on their latest visits to Riley

Hospital. "Mary had braces fitted on both legs and is learning to use a small set of crutches at physical therapy. We take her to PT twice a week in Glen Falls at the hospital. She tested normal on mental and other developmental skills, and we're proud of her." Katy turned a mock glare at Michael. "My only objection to her treatment is that she still prefers him to me during PT. She doesn't want Michael out of her sight while the therapist works with her."

Michael just beamed in response. "It's just my natural charm. I can't help that."

"Oh, you!" Katy handed Mary to Michael and retrieved Ruth from his lap. "Our little Ruthie is making progress as well. She's delayed a few months but starting to catch up with developmental skills. My sweet revenge is that she wants me there during therapy, not Sir Michael." She smirked, and he winked at me.

Donna helped me finish examining little Robert, then left to retrieve the vaccinations for each child.

After making brief notes to finish later because of the busy day, I excused myself to go to the next visit. Michael extended a firm handshake. "Thanks for all you do for us. We appreciate it more than you'll ever know."

"Quite all right, my friend. It's good to see the family healthy and progressing."

"One more thing, Doc. I saw my good friend Jack O'Conner arrive at the office when Donna brought us back. He's been by my side through all the trials we've experienced in the past. How's he doing?"

"Well…" I hesitated. "He's out of the hospital, as you can see. I can't tell you much more than what you already know because of patient confidentiality. Talk to him before you leave. His medical problems haven't killed his zest for life, and he loves talking. He should be the next postmaster in my opinion. Then he could spend more time talking than walking."

Michael grinned. "Yeah. Maybe he should run for mayor when he recovers. That would really suit him. I'm all in for promoting that idea."

DONNA GOT my attention as I left the room. "You'd better go look at Johnny Morton. Christine finally got him to sit down in the back room and soak his hand. He's pasty white, sweating, and sick at his stomach. I'll be with you as soon as I give the kids their shots."

Muttering to myself, I rushed to the lab and treatment area. Our aspiring fisherman indeed looked ill. "Hey, Johnny. What have you done to yourself now?"

"Please, Doc. Don't ask. I'm not feelin' so good. I think I'm gonna pass out." With those words, Johnny keeled over onto the floor, dumping a full wash basin of water with Betadine soap all over himself while thoroughly drenching Christine, the cabinets, and the floor.

Christine screamed as she lost her balance trying to hold on to him and sat down hard on the floor beside Johnny's prostrate form. She had somehow eased him down gently.

I ran to check Johnny, squatted, and log-rolled him carefully onto his side, all the while trying to keep my pants out of the yellow-brown cesspool on the floor. "Impressive save, Christine. He didn't even bump his head with you supporting him on the way down."

Donna arrived with the smelling salts and thrust them under his nose as he lay stretched out in the lab. Within seconds, he pushed the bottle of ammonia salts away and tried to sit up, showering more of the room and the three of us with the nasty soapy water.

Christine got to her feet on the second try, after first sliding in the liquid and sitting back down hard. She cast an accusing glance my way, tearing up and flushed with embarrassment. "Just look at my clothes. Ruined! Once a perfectly fitting new blue dress. Covered with this slop. How will I face the patients? This is mortifying. The cleaning bill will be enormous if anything is salvageable. What's a poor working girl to do?"

Donna whispered, "She certainly hasn't lost her gift of gab. From what I can see, all our clothes are stained with yellow-brown splotches. The patients will love it."

Johnny looked up, an innocent expression on his countenance. "I'm so sorry. I must've passed out. Did I dump the basin on the floor?"

Donna nodded. "On the floor, on Christine, and now on us. Thank you very much!"

Christine's eyes continued to water. "Everybody stop staring at me. Sure, I shed a few tears over my ruined clothes, but this stuff burns my eyes. Excuse me while I use a different sink to rinse my face and eyes before I go blind."

With a loud sigh, I extended my hand to help Johnny off the floor after determining that he had no fresh injuries from his syncopal spell. His hand bled more after getting back in the chair, requiring a temporary pressure dressing. His lure had fallen out on the floor, and the remaining hook in his hand required minimal effort to remove.

Donna finished checking his BP and pulse. "You're back to normal, but I still don't trust you."

"If you feel faint still, we'll put you in room 1 to lie down for a while."

"No, thanks, Doc. I'm fine now. Sorry to be so much trouble. I'll make it up to you. I'll cut your grass for free the rest of the summer and bring fresh fish for the ladies to enjoy."

"Not necessary. Just warn us next time you feel like fainting."

Christine returned from the bathroom sink looking liked a half-drowned, muddy kitten. She kept trying to smooth her clothes down as she sorrowfully assessed her new dress.

"Don't worry, Christine. The office will cover the cleaning bill and the purchase of a comparable new outfit," I told her.

"Does that offer apply to the nurse too?" Donna asked.

"It definitely is an offer for all staff members." I shook my head, pretending remorse. "I'm afraid it doesn't apply to the perpetrator, however."

"You mean me?" Johnny asked. "Am I the perpetrator?"

Assuming my most solemn look, I nodded. "You are."

"Aw, I don't want anything but my hand fixed and my lure back. I'm sorry. Let me help mop up the floor." He got up and immediately slipped on the wet tiles.

Christine grabbed his arm and pointed at the chair. "Sit! Don't get up until I tell you."

He looked so pitiful, and Christine so flustered, that Donna chuckled. I could no longer restrain myself and joined in the ever-increasing volume of laughter.

Christine stared at us. "What?"

That only amplified our merriment. She scowled and made faces as we laughed uncontrollably, and Johnny joined in the fun with loud guffaws. Finally, Christine started to laugh too.

Interrupted by a knock on the door, we attempted a measure of self-control. I glanced over to see Art McKay, funeral director, emergency service provider, and coroner, peeking around the corner as he held the door open. "Anyone hurt? Sounded like someone got killed back here until you all started laughing."

"Thanks for checking. Other than Johnny's sore hand, the only injury is to our self-esteem. We're all a mess."

Art shook his head, trying not to laugh. "Anything I can do?"

"Yes. There are spare long white coats in the closet at the end of the hallway. If you could get three of them for us, at least we can cover up some of the damage."

"You know what will happen, don't you? The gossip column in the town newspaper will be all over this. May take you a bit to live it down." Art covered his mouth, suppressing his laughter. After recovering, he said, "I'll get the coats for you. Just a second."

Christine wilted into a chair she pulled out. "Do I have to go out there and face our patients?"

"I'm sorry, but you do. I have an idea though. Tell them there's a necessary time delay while we clean up and sterilize the area. There are flecks and splotches of blood all over the floor and cabinet. We were fortunately splashed with mostly soapy water. Give everyone an opportunity to reschedule later today or tomorrow. I'll order food out at five, and we'll work late to catch up. Meanwhile, if you want to call the downtown ladies' shop, I'll start with buying whatever clothing you order for this afternoon. Let's take a break until after lunch unless there's another emergency sitting in the waiting room. On second thought, see what Jack wants to do. I'll go ahead with his visit now if he prefers."

Donna spoke up. "No genuine emergencies now. Mainly routine appointments. I'll check with Jack. Come on, Christine. Let's go make the announcements."

Still smiling, Art distributed the white coats and took a bow to a round of applause.

CHAPTER 14—END OF A LONG DAY

*A*fter the fiasco and delay because of Johnny's fishing accident, the patients all elected to reschedule, most for later in the day. By 11:30, we had the mess cleaned up but were exhausted with the workday just beginning. I slumped in a chair in the waiting room, mopping my forehead. "I believe I got all the blood stains out of the carpet. How is the clean-up progressing in the back room?"

Christine stood in the hallway, haggard, bedraggled, and undecided about what to accomplish next. "You need to add combat and hazardous duty pay to your employees' compensation. Not to mention uniform expense reimbursement."

"Did Geraldine have clothing in your sizes to deliver from her shop?"

Donna joined us, collapsing in a chair across the room. "Supposedly. I hope she hurries. I'm miserable in these damp, stained clothes."

Seated by the picture window, I turned to see who had pulled into our parking lot. "Exciting news, ladies. Barry House is here to deliver our lunch. You have your choice of cheeseburgers, a works pizza, or both. It's the least I can do."

Barry knocked as he opened the front door. "Service with a laugh. Sorry. I mean smile. Brought your lunch with all the fixings. I had to see this for myself. Connie Thorndike, my favorite hypochondriac, told me all the lurid details."

I motioned him into the waiting room. "Wipe that silly grin off your face and have a seat. And you're not sorry. I'm anxious to hear her version of the story. It has to be over the top."

"Where do you want me to set the food?"

Donna relieved Barry of the sacks of burgers and boxed pizza. "I'll take these to the break room. We sure appreciate getting this. I'm famished."

"Christine, please pay Barry out of the petty cash drawer. I'll replace it with a personal check later. Feel free to grab Diet Cokes out of my stash in the refrigerator. Enjoy your meal. I want to hear Connie's version of our brush with death this morning. I'll watch for Geraldine's car, so relax if you can."

Barry took a seat nearby with a smirk on his face. "Well, it's a remarkable tale, Doc. It seems that Johnny Morton caught a twenty-five-pound bass that nearly bit his arm off, and your office staff made light of his injury. He had to wait an hour for treatment and passed out from blood loss before you finally got to him. She plans to advise him to see her lawyer. Not that she wishes you any harm, mind you. Just looking after Johnny."

"Did Johnny tell her that whopper?"

"No, he didn't. I asked her, but she has it from a 'reliable witness.'"

I pursed my lips and blew out a loud breath. "Whew! She is trying out for an Oscar. Such ridiculous baloney. She wasn't even here."

Barry laughed. "Don't take it too hard. You're in most understanding company. She's been spreading rumors all over town that my store is overrun with cockroaches and rats. Told anyone who would listen that our lunch wasn't fit for consumption. She had the unmitigated gall to trumpet that fabrication while eating our special at the counter today. Ethel was furious, but I assured her that Connie is harmless. No one believes a word she says anymore. Just inexpensive entertainment."

"Thank goodness for that small favor."

"I wouldn't worry about it. She's a poor lonely soul looking for attention. Doesn't believe a word of her own claptrap from my observation. Got up and told Ethel how delicious the meal was and gave her a generous tip. Left Ethel flabbergasted. She doesn't know Connie as you and I do."

"Well, she'll learn. She does us the same way. Complains about the wait time, service, and treatment. Then smiles and blows kisses to the staff while she offers profuse thanks for the wonderful medical care. She always makes sure everyone in the waiting room hears her say she wouldn't use another doctor, as she leaves. She's too much, but you can't really stay upset with her. Like you said, inexpensive entertainment."

Barry glanced around the room. "Looks like you're all set up to start again after lunch. Everything's back in order. Will you be working late this evening? We close at eight, but I'll extend the hours for any prescriptions if needed."

"The girls will keep you informed. Thanks for your support. And I needed a good laugh. Thanks for the story."

Barry stood to leave. "Looks like Geraldine just pulled in. I'll be going. Let me know if there's anything else I can do to help."

"Thanks for being a friend. On days like this, we need one."

Barry held the door for Geraldine, then left, laughing, as he pulled out his car keys.

"Just a second, I'll get the ladies from the back," I said. "They're most eager to see you. I'll give you a check for their new clothing since one of our patients ruined theirs." Then I called, "Ladies, Geraldine's here and has your order. I'll grab a sandwich to eat on the way home. I want to change too, while there's still time before patients arrive for afternoon appointments. Lock the office, change clothes, and relax a few minutes. We start again at one and I'll be back about then."

Christine rushed back to the waiting room, clapping her hands. "This may turn out better than I thought. New clothes. Lunch is delicious. What more can a girl ask for?"

Donna joined her. "Yes. Thanks for providing the lunch and new clothing. It wasn't your fault or responsibility to pay for everything."

"Glad to do it. Need to keep valuable help happy and satisfied. See you in a little over an hour. Chalk it up to a pay bonus for hazardous duty." Scooping up a sandwich and drink, I hurried to my car.

~

DONNA HANDED me the first chart for the afternoon. "Jack's back for his appointment, and he can't stop laughing about this morning. You're the talk of the town today, Doc. He wants to hear your version of the disaster that's assuming ever-increasing proportion all over Glen Oaks."

"That's privileged patient information. I can't do that."

"The patients will all be asking today. Seems you're quite the celebrity after saving Johnny from the jaws of death."

"Did he actually say that?"

"Why, yes, he did. Don't make light of it. While you did CPR, we kept Johnny breathing until Art McKay got here with the ambulance to transport the poor boy to the hospital. You see, Christine and I are basking in the afterglow of our victory in the life-and-death battle to save our patient this morning." Her serious demeanor dissolved as she burst out laughing.

I was speechless.

"What? You don't believe me? Just ask Jack. He had it from Janie, who had it from Ann Kilgore, who had it from—"

"Never mind. I get your point. We will put a stop to this nonsense right now. Just sweetly inform the others that patient confidentiality prohibits our further discussion of this matter. They want information? Talk to Johnny."

"I hate to burst your bubble, but Johnny's laying it on thick, enjoying the notoriety."

I shook my head. "This is definitely a no-win situation for the practice."

"Not at all, Doc. You'd pay a lot of hard-earned money for publicity like this. The phone's been ringing off the wall. Seems everyone wants an appointment. Several new people called in, laughing and asking to see you. Word's got around that you provide entertainment along with the medical practice. Much more interesting than most other doctors in the county. So get over it and go see Jack."

$$\sim$$

JACK LOOKED great as I entered exam room 1. He stood and offered a firm handshake, smiling and relaxed. "Doc, you have the most interesting practice in the county. Did Donna tell you all the wild tales making the rounds?"

Why did these episodes get so blown out of proportion? "Yes, unfortunately. I heard unbelievable exaggerations from several sources. Sorry. I can't divulge any information because of patient confidentiality. You must ask Johnny what happened. I'm sure he'll be glad to enlighten you with the gory details, especially regarding the bass he caught."

Jack sat down, chuckling. "I don't expect you to give me any information about Johnny. He doesn't need any help to spread the tall tales all over town—singing your praises, by the way. He gave me his 'version number seven,' from what I could find out from some of my friends."

Finally relaxed, I took a seat to review and update the chart. "You look great today. Healthy color. No distress. I'm amazed."

"Looks are not deceiving in this case. I feel wonderful, thanks to an efficient hospital staff and my doctors. I told you I'm not ready to die yet. Got too much to accomplish first."

I raised my eyebrows.

"Don't look at me that way. I'm ready to meet my Maker, just not too soon. I plan to beat this cancer. At least for a while. I know it may come back with a vengeance, but not until my time is up. Got to see my daughter married and graduated from med school first. Also need to see

95

William settled spiritually. I fully believe that God will at least give me that much time to live."

"I trust He will do that. You're not lacking in faith, that's for sure."

"I'm immortal until He's finished with me in this life. Then I'm ready to be genuinely immortal in the forever of God's tomorrow."

I placed my hand on his knee. "I'm glad you've found such peace with this, my friend."

"Enough of this maudlin discussion about death and dying. I'm planning for life. When can I start chemotherapy, or whatever treatment regimen Doc Stanberry has in mind."

Following a detailed examination, Jack got up from the exam table without help and tucked his shirt back into his slacks. "What do you think?"

"I think you look great. Your last protime was normal. There's no sign of more blood clots. No evidence of bleeding because of anticoagulation. No abnormality on the physical exam. When do you see Dr. Stanberry for follow-up?"

"Next Tuesday."

"We'll leave it up to his expert advice. Usually about six weeks after surgery in the absence of other complications. Unfortunately, the pulmonary embolus set you back, but you appear fully recovered from that complication. It's his call now. However, I expect he'll want you starting treatment as soon as possible. From my reading between the lines of his last consultation note, the one dictated the day before we discharged you from the hospital, that's the gist of his thoughts."

"I'm as ready as anyone could ever be. Thanks again. And now, to find my buddy Johnny. I want to hear the newest version of his out-of-body experience. One more thing before I leave. The bizarre antics and entertainment this morning did me a world of good. I feel so much better. Laughter is a good medicine, just like the Bible says."

Jack made his way to see Christine for his exit paperwork, laughing all the way.

AT 9:15 THAT NIGHT, the last patient departed for Barry House's pharmacy. True to his word, Barry patiently awaited our last appointment. Donna had called the prescription in to expedite matters in view of his courtesy.

Christine busied herself collecting trash while Donna straightened up the furniture in the exam rooms, taking time to resupply material used up during the office visits.

Streetlights had come on several minutes ago, as dusk descended over Glen Oaks, our sleepy, beloved, nosy town. Sitting at the table in the break room finishing the last charts, I wanted nothing more than to get home myself. I hurriedly added the finishing touches to my notes and carried the charts to Christine's desk for filing in the morning.

The ladies stood by the door, ready to leave, worn down from the long but eventful day. Christine waved. "Goodnight, Doc. Thanks for lunch and for replacing our destroyed clothing. One thing about working for you, it is never routine or boring, at least not for long."

Donna looked thoughtful. "For once, I agree with Christine. Thanks for everything, and it's not in the least a dull job. I can't say I enjoyed every minute, but I'm certain we'll all enjoy the afterglow as Johnny spreads rumors and sings our praises around the county. Ever think of adding him to the payroll? He'd make a brilliant publicity manager."

"No doubt about that, but no. I'm not hiring him. I'd be prematurely gray-headed with him underfoot all the time. Have a good evening, short perhaps, but hopefully restful. I'll finish locking up and take the bank deposit to the drop box. See you both in the morning. Drive safe."

I relaxed during my short trip home. Another action-packed day chalked up in the charming town of Glen Oaks.

CHAPTER 15—HOLIDAY HOUSE CALL

*B*y Labor Day, September 5, 1977, the office had settled into a normal routine once more, thankfully minus most of the excitement brought on by my favorite fisherman, Johnny Morton. Relieved to have a day off, I planned early morning rounds at the hospital so I could enjoy my time off with Janet, our children, and our extended family. Hot dogs and hamburgers for grilling awaited me. Deck chairs for the adults. Backyard swing set, tricycles, and sandbox for the youngsters. What better holiday could one hope for?

When I arrived at the hospital at 6:45 a.m. and parked my car in the doctors' lot, I switched off the ignition and stepped out into a refreshing balmy breeze, the temperature just climbing to seventy with comfortable conditions expected to last into the evening hours. Stars faded in the eastern sky as sunrise approached at 7:15, with light pink-tinged gray cumulus clouds floating across the horizon, already visible. I inhaled deeply, savoring the scent of honeysuckle growing wild at the rear of the hospital property. With the omens all favorable, I hurried to see my patients.

Pleasantly surprised, I finished rounds in an hour without interruption from the emergency room. Feeling great, I hurried to the car, enjoying the caroling of a single robin in an oak tree on the hospital grounds. Several of his fellow travelers had already gone to find a place to winter in the deep woods or at points far south of Indiana. The rest would soon follow them. I missed the full-throated springtime chorus of multitudes of his fellows but felt grateful for the joyful little guy singing *cheer-up, cheerily* for me. According to one almanac, we could expect bitter cold and blowing snow in the not too distant future. Not a pleasant thought!

Once again home, I grabbed the *Glen Oaks News* from the delivery box, retrieved a cup of hot coffee, and settled on the porch swing to keep up with community events and newsmakers. Janet had the kids up, and breakfast would soon be ready. Pancakes with hot maple syrup, fresh strawberries generously applied, all topped off with whipped cream, a gourmet's delight, had my salivary glands working overtime just inhaling the wonderful scent from the kitchen.

One of the most troublesome problems I faced in private solo practice continued to plague me as I yearned to develop the coveted art of complete mental relaxation. Ominously, I couldn't shake the conviction that our family gathering had a built-in interruption evolving. I had delivered a baby on about every holiday in the year. Why would this day be any different? I shifted uneasily on the swing.

Relieved when Janet announced that breakfast was ready, I folded my paper, downed the last of my coffee, and took my place at the head of the table, next to the wall phone, naturally. All my patients had my home telephone number and few hesitated to use it.

Our children had learned simple prayers of thanks in Sunday school and loved taking turns saying thanks before our meals. Cindy claimed the privilege as she solemnly offered grace. "God is great, God is good. Now we thank Him for our food. Amen!" The twins applauded, and the meal began as Janet saw that each child had a fair share of the delicious breakfast.

～

I FINISHED MY MEAL, relished a frosty glass of milk, and downed my third cup of Folger's medium blend before the first call of the day. My wife had the children out at their playground as I continued sitting at the table, attempting to come to terms with anxiety over the day. Startled, I nearly tipped over my fourth cup of coffee when the loud ringing shattered the quiet peace of the morning. I jerked the phone from the wall mount hook. "Hello, who's calling please?" I tried to sound calm and cordial.

Words spilled out in a torrent of rapid-fire speech. "Morning, Doc. It's Art McKay. Got called out on an emergency run a few minutes ago. Picked up Ollie Stone, and Willie Robertson is on the way. We're at the Isaac home with Matilda. She called about her mother, Lydia, at nine thirty." Grossly obese, Art paused to get his breath, huffing and puffing. A sure sign he had been running with the Stryker transport stretcher after sliding it out of the bed of the ambulance, which was, in reality, one of his retooled hearses.

His health concerned me a lot. "Slow down and get your breath Art. You won't be able to help anybody if you collapse from overexertion. First rule: take care of yourself so you can continue the rescue effort."

Pausing briefly, Art did his best to regain control. "Sorry. I know better. Just can't seem to help myself when there's a crisis."

"It's okay. You're a caring man. Please go ahead with your report."

Art resumed the conversation with an obvious attempt to moderate his speech. "Matilda found Lydia passed out on the kitchen floor this morning. Checked a glucometer reading to rule out hypoglycemia. Blood glucose 185. Ollie's checking her over now for signs of injury or stroke."

"Be sure and watch him. He's not too experienced." Ollie loved the excitement of emergency care and frequently engaged in hyperbole and histrionics.

Ollie's excitement came over the phone loud and clear in his panicked sing-song voice. "Art, get over here. I think she may be dead already."

I shuddered as Art dropped their phone, yelling for Ollie to get out of the way.

Terrified about what was happening, I tried yelling into my phone to get someone to answer. "Willie, are you there yet?"

No answer. Background shrieks, probably Matilda and Ollie.

"Anybody. Someone. Pick up the phone. Let me know what's happening."

Still nothing but the sound of pandemonium.

Disgusted now, I slammed the phone back on the hook, grabbed my stethoscope off the wall peg, and ran to my car. The Isaac home was only five minutes away, two minutes the way I would drive today. Jumping in, I quickly started the engine, remembered to yell that I had an emergency, and saw the disappointment on my wife's face as I backed into the street and took off in a cloud of dust.

During the quick drive to the Isaac home, I reviewed all I knew about Lydia: elderly, diabetic, hypertensive, enlarged heart, poor compliance with medications, known to pass out whenever she had an audience, a real character. On the positive side of the scale: sweet, polite, concerned about others, and a gentle spirit. She and Matilda cared for frail Mr. Isaac. Why did people have to be so complicated?

Skidding to a stop in their gravel driveway behind the ambulance, I heard pebbles bouncing off the street behind me. I grabbed my stethoscope, breathless myself, and ran up the steps to the front porch.

The interior of the Isaac home was familiar. I had been a frequent visitor for house calls over the last few years. A crowd hovered around Lydia still lying on the kitchen floor beside the breakfast bar, just visible through the doorway. I charged through the living room and dining room to join the would-be caretakers in the kitchen.

Willie Robertson, forty-nine-year-old EMT, levelheaded and calm, had come on the scene bringing a measure of sanity and order to the chaotic situation. He knelt beside Lydia as Art bent over, rechecking her vital signs. Young Ollie Stone, looking not at all chastened, sat rocking back and forth on both knees in the corner of the room where Willie had ordered his retreat.

Willie looked up at me and winked. "How're you doing, Doc? Sorry we didn't get to answer you on the phone. I heard you yelling but had my hands full." The phone receiver still dangled down the wall, the cord stretched out nearly straight, a buzzing dial tone sounding continually. I replaced the phone on the receiver to kill the noise.

Not sure whether to laugh or cry, I stood silently considering my options. Retreat? Go out and come back in calmly? Lecture Ollie about his obvious hysterical reaction? Pretend it's only another normal day in Glen Oaks? The last option appealed most to me. "Would you be so kind as to fill me in on the details?"

Everyone spoke at once until I held up my hands. "Please, folks. I appreciate all the valuable help, but I want to start off with Willie's narrative."

No one appeared offended. Art pulled out a chair and sat down, wiping sweat from his brow with an over-sized red bandana handkerchief pulled from his pocket. Ollie got up, eyeing the bowl of fruit sitting on the counter. I watched as he surreptitiously picked up a banana and peeled it, glancing furtively around the room.

Matilda noticed him as she pulled out a chair for herself. "It's okay, Ollie. Help yourself. That's what they're for. I just appreciate your rapid response when we need you."

I stood watching as Lydia ever so slowly turned her head toward me, fluttering her eyelids before finally opening them fully. "Why, hello, Doctor. I didn't expect to see you here on your day off. It's a holiday, isn't it?"

Doing my best not to laugh out loud, I mentally listed another of her quirks. An unparalleled master in the art of understatement.

Willie coughed and cleared his throat. "Doc, it seems that Lydia got up feeling well until she came to fix breakfast. Matilda heard her hit the floor, jumped out of bed, and came running to find her unconscious and jerking her arms and legs for about a minute. She called Art and tried to do CPR until Lydia revived enough to push her away from her chest. So Matilda backed off and Lydia went limp. That's how she presented when the boys first got here."

Willie took a long breath. "Unfortunately, Ollie thought she had passed when he couldn't feel her radial pulse right away. He didn't notice that she was breathing, and his reaction caused quite a ruckus. Don't worry about it. We'll have a training session at the ambulance barn as soon as we get back."

"That we will," Art said. "Ollie meant well but didn't read the situation right."

"I'm sure you'll take care of the details. Let's get back to Lydia. What are you finding? Any injuries? Any focal weakness of the extremities?"

Willie continued with his oral report. "Level of consciousness returning to normal. No head, neck, or pelvic tenderness to palpation. No apparent carotid bruits in the neck."

Pulling out a chair, I relaxed for the first time since entering the home, my emotions under control at last. I smiled and nodded for Willie to continue. This boy was learning his job!

"We haven't tried to move her yet, but she's moving her arms and legs normally. Her heart and lungs, at least from this angle, sound clear and steady. Maybe a simple syncopal episode? Would you like to check on her now before we try moving her off the floor?"

Lydia grunted and turned over on her right side. "Not necessary. I'm fine now. Help me up."

She moved so fast that Willie and Art had no time to restrain her. She agilely got up on her knees as she steadied herself with her hands placed on the kitchen tiles.

I got out of my chair. "Slow down. They need to finish the assessment and help you get up the first time."

Lydia made a face. "Oh, phooey with that. I'm getting stiff down here. If no one will give me a hand, I'll just get up by myself."

Art rolled his eyes and shrugged. "Wait a second. I'll help you if it's okay with Doc."

Nodding for him to proceed, I stifled another chuckle.

Once back on her feet, Lydia insisted on retiring to the living room where her big, soft green La-Z-Boy recliner sat in one corner. Ollie tossed his second banana peel in the kitchen trash can and hurried to offer his right arm while patting the back of her hand with his left as she clung to his proffered arm. In a lot of ways, they were much alike. Histrionic. Hilarious. Ham-actors and loveable.

My examination completed, I shook hands with Matilda after she walked me to the door. "Make an appointment this week for your mom."

"Don't worry about that. I think Ollie might have been right. It looked to me like mom had died. Still not sure she didn't. Maybe the boys brought her back. Anyway, she'll be in your office tomorrow."

Poor, overworked, gullible Matilda. "That'll be fine. Always glad to see you in the office." I hoped she caught my emphasis on the word *office*. Feeling a little guilty, I hastily added, "Call me if you have questions or if she has any more attacks." But I sure wouldn't break the speed limit getting there.

Matilda teared up, unable to comment further as she held the door open for the boys to wheel out the still-empty Stryker stretcher.

After exchanging pleasantries with Art, I motioned for Willie to join us. "Be sure and talk to Ollie about his tendency to engage in loud, upsetting outbursts. We all know he means well, but he detracts from your overall service to the community with his uncontrolled behavior."

Art nodded. "Don't worry. We'll both talk with him and go over protocols for calmly doing his job. He tries too hard sometimes. I can't help but feel sorry for him."

Willie stood behind Art with a twisted grin on his face. "We'll take care of it. He's bound to get better." Left unsaid: How could he be any worse?

Ollie opened the passenger door of the ambulance and leaned out. "You fellas coming? I'm getting hungry."

Willie threw his hands up. "He's hungry. I haven't even had breakfast yet. He ate two bananas in there and grabbed a chocolate chip cookie to go on the way out the door. I give up! Come on, Art. We need to have a long talk with that boy."

~

RELAXING with a much slower drive home, I reviewed my holiday so far. For sure, just another "normal" day in Glen Oaks. An elderly patient who loved attention, willing to go to any extent to get it, especially on notable days of the year: any holiday, first day at the county fair, downtown parades, anywhere a crowd might gather.

My family and guests would never believe my story. Thankfully, there was such a thing as patient confidentiality. I couldn't share with my wife until everyone went home today. And the day was still early enough that anything could happen.

CHAPTER 16—SPECIAL HONORS

*T*uesday, September 6, dawned with leaden-gray skies, a brisk cool breeze out of the southwest, and frequent rain showers. On entering the hospital, I shook my umbrella and sent rain droplets cascading onto the rubber mat inside the doctors' entrance, then proceeded to the first-floor conference room at the far end of the building.

The monthly staff meeting, deferred one day from the usual Monday meeting because of the holiday, was scheduled to begin in five minutes at 7:00 a.m. In my left hand, I carried the folder with the report from the scholarship committee regarding the four candidates. Two had gained the recommendation of the entire committee of seven members but required a full staff vote to formalize the decision.

After grabbing a cup of coffee, a steaming plate of scrambled eggs, breakfast rolls slathered with butter, and crisp bacon served by the dietary staff outside the conference room, I took a seat near the head of the table, waiting my turn as secretary of the scholarship committee to read the report. Smiling, I considered my meal. It might not pass muster with the American Heart Association, but it sure filled the bill for this gathering of hard-working rural town and country doctors.

Chief-of-Staff Dr. Bill Johnson banged his gavel on the podium, hushing the small talk around the long conference table seating twenty-five physicians. "The meeting will now come to order. Dr. Langley, secretary of the medical staff, will now read the minutes from our last meeting, Monday, August 1, 1977."

Doc Langley carried his notes to the podium while Bill sat down to his left and began sipping his coffee and sampling the delicious breakfast. At seventy-five, Doc Langley continued to practice medicine in a rural town, dividing his time between seeing patients in the office in the morning, making house calls in the afternoon, and continuing to perform minor surgeries at the hospital.

Only half listening to his sonorous voice reciting the boring but necessary details of last month's meeting, which I had already reviewed at length, I enjoyed my food and the camaraderie of our shared experiences. Then came the motion to accept the minutes, and I raised my hand in favor and gathered up my papers as the motion was adopted.

Bill nodded for me to proceed with the committee recommendations. Taking my turn at the podium, I pulled out the first application. "Several of you know the first candidate, Lynn O'Conner, one of my patients who has worked with several of you as a student observer this summer. She's interested in a career as a medical doctor. Lynn has a 4.0 GPA at Indiana University with two years of pre-med completed. She meets the academic requirement set by the sponsor of the scholarship program. In addition, her father is disabled with gastric carcinoma and has an uncertain prognosis. He has provided her support until this illness. Now the family needs help if Lynn is to continue pursuing her dream. He and Lynn have filed the papers showing the need."

Taking a sip of water, I felt pleased at sensing the sympathetic mood of the staff. Most knew her and her quality of dedication. "The scholarship committee voted unanimously, all seven members being present, to offer Lynn O'Conner a one-year full scholarship for her third year at Indiana University in pre-medical studies. She plans to apply for acceptance at Indiana University School of Medicine after completing the third year of undergraduate studies. The School of Medicine continues to offer slots to outstanding students after completion of three years of study. Therefore, the committee proposes to offer her a full four-year scholarship for medical school, conditional on her acceptance to the medical college along with continuing satisfactory academic achievement. Finally, she has signified her willingness to return to this local community to practice medicine for at least the next three years following internship and residency." I set the folder down on the podium and glanced around. "Questions? Comments?"

Fred Howard, staff pathologist, raised a point. "I assume she is planning on primary care. Is that the case?"

Rob Hendrick nodded. "She wants to become a family doctor. I interviewed Lynn for the committee. That's her number one goal. She's already affixed her signature to the section regarding her promise to practice in the local county."

Jerome Hayden, our chief of emergency medicine, raised his hand. "What happens if she decides not to practice here after training? That would sure be a waste of scholarship dollars." Leave it to him to throw in a monkey wrench.

Rob, chairman of the scholarship committee, glanced my way. "Do you mind if I continue fielding questions, Carl?"

"Not at all. I want everyone to feel comfortable with the decision of the committee. Lynn is my patient, but I don't want to seem to inappropriately favor her selection for top honors."

Bill chuckled. "No one suspects your motives, Carl. Please continue with your line of thought, Rob."

Rob stood and came to the podium. I handed him the folder as I returned to my coffee. "As part of the agreement, the applicant has to agree to repay the scholarship fund in full within three years of training if the contract to return is not fulfilled. The hospital attorney and the benefactor of the scholarship have signed off on the paperwork. The committee expects no problems."

"She's a fine young lady from a responsible local family," Doc Langley interjected. "Her father has delivered my mail for years. He's the salt of the earth, a most exemplary man with a wonderful family, all very deserving. She has my vote of confidence."

Jerome nodded. "Sounds good to me. I just wanted to be certain. You know."

Rob cleared his throat. "If there is no further discussion, with Dr. Johnson's permission, I would like to move that we accept the recommendation of the full committee."

Bill Johnson assumed the podium again. "Permission granted. Is there a second to the motion?"

In less than a minute, the motion had a second and carried unanimously. I then presented the second committee recommendation regarding Paul Hawley, another deserving student, a twenty-two-year-old Summa Cum Laude graduate from Purdue University, already accepted by the Indiana University School of Medicine for the fall semester, also in need of financial help. I didn't know Paul since he came from the far western corner of the county, but I enthusiastically added my assent to the committee report. The medical staff soon added his name to the roster, and we had our scholarships set for the year.

Bill Johnson worked hard at keeping the meeting on time and brought things to a conclusion in another half hour. "We all have patients to care for and busy schedules to attend to, but before we go, I have a surprise for the medical staff. After reviewing the committee recommendations with Dr. Hendrick over the weekend, I knew that we had our first two candidates."

Bill motioned to Ann Kilgore standing outside the open door. Today, Ann worked in her official position as nursing supervisor for the day shift. "Please bring our guests in so I can introduce them to the staff."

Ann gave a radiant smile and stood aside, holding out her left arm to invite Lynn O'Conner and Paul Hawley to precede her into the conference room. Lynn, blond with big brown eyes and a vivacious smile, blushed as she walked to the podium to shake hands with Dr. Johnson and acknowledge the warm applause from the staff. She was followed closely by a handsome, blue-eyed, athletic youth with dark brown hair, Paul Hawley.

After the formal presentation by Dr. Johnson, the staff gave another prolonged round of applause along with a standing ovation, much to the embarrassment of the two young people. They appeared tremendously relieved when Ann Kilgore rescued them from the unexpected attention.

Ann waited for the commotion to subside, then said, "You've taken enough of their time. They're all mine now, and the *Glen Falls Daily News* is here to take pictures of our first scholarship recipients for the morning edition of tomorrow's paper."

As the meeting broke up, Rob joined Bill and me at the head of the table. "Those two are certainly photogenic. They would make a great-looking couple. I wouldn't be surprised if the committee is accused of playing at match-making."

Bill grinned as he slapped Rob on the back. "From their shared discrete smiles at one another, along with frequent furtive eye contact, I'd say the charge might have a certain merit. Remember the days when we got our assignments in the internship and residency match program following med school? Looks to me like you fellas are into another kind of match-making altogether."

Rob laughed. "I wouldn't mind that at all. They're both talented kids. I've had the privilege to work with both of them during the summer. The staff won't regret awarding them these scholarships. If something more comes of it, I'll be happy for them. Those kids have sacrificed and nearly exhausted themselves working toward their dreams. I'd be happy to see them share the journey as a couple. Wouldn't you?"

Bill nodded. "I sure would. We may have set a precedence for the future. Our motto: Find happiness at our hospital. Win a scholarship and discover your true love." He walked off laughing uproariously at his own joke.

~

As I parked behind the office at 10:30, I saw Christine standing beside the picture window sipping coffee and watching for my arrival.

She opened the back door for me as I approached, head cocked and a smile on her face. "Welcome. My favorite doctor has arrived. We have about ten minutes before the first patient, and no one is here yet other than Donna and me." She pulled out a chair at the lounge table as she hastened to pour a cup of coffee for my enjoyment. "Sit down a few minutes and enjoy. Would you like to sample my holiday chocolate cake?"

"Sure. Why not?" I tasted my coffee while she cut a generous piece of chocolate cake with fudge icing. "What gives with the red-carpet treatment today? I know the wheels in your devious brain are spinning at an unfathomable velocity. There has to be a catch somewhere."

She smirked. "Why, Doctor. You should have more faith in me. Would I ever use bribery or practice deceit?"

Wrinkling up my brows, I opened my mouth to respond.

"On second thought, don't answer that." She placed her right index finger over her lips, interrupting me.

Donna sat on the other side of the room on a bar stool, calibrating the lab equipment for the day to prepare for running blood tests. She pivoted about to face us. "Don't be fooled by her. She's been fretting for the last hour about the scholarship awards. She has proposed three or four elaborate schemes to weasel the news from you about the winners. I told her to just ask. I'm sure you'll satisfy her insatiable curiosity once again."

Time to tease a little. "I'll tell you all about it during our noon break. The recipients will be featured in the newspapers tomorrow. Very worthy students." Pushing my chair back as if to stand, I gave up my charade, unable to keep from laughing at her crestfallen expression.

Donna wrinkled her nose as she swiveled her seat back around to finish setting up the lab equipment. "Humph! You're making her worse, Doc. Curiosity will be responsible for her untimely demise someday.

Tell her to get back to work." She looked over her shoulder to wink at me, not meaning a word of what she'd said.

I leaned forward, folded my hands on the table, and motioned for Christine to have a seat across from me. "Might as well get this over with. You'll not give me a moment of peace until you have all the facts. Right?"

Unembarrassed, Christine beamed. "Oh, you're so right. I have to know about Lynn. Did she get one of the scholarships?"

Donna finished her task and joined us, taking a seat beside Christine. She intertwined her fingers, elbows propped up on the table, and leaned her chin on her hands. "Honestly, I'm dying for the news too. I simply refuse to use subterfuge. Not like a certain person I could name." She leaned over and gently nudged Christine's shoulder.

Not at all taken aback, Christine said, "Please get on with it. I won't be able to concentrate on my job until I know about Lynn."

Taking a few minutes, I laid out the details of the awards given to Lynn O'Conner and Paul Hawley as the ladies sat in rapt silence. I even mentioned the interest shown by the subtle body language exchanged between the two young people, knowing they would appreciate it.

Christine sighed. "How romantic. I think I'm going to cry." She grabbed a tissue from the box on the end of the table and wiped her eyes. "What color did Lynn wear for the ceremony?"

My chair scraped on the linoleum as I pushed it back and stood up. "Christine, get a grip. I don't pay attention to such details. We celebrated scholarship awards, not a wedding."

"Leave it to her!" Donna exclaimed. "Ready to cry over something that may never happen."

Christine shrugged. "I don't care what you think. You have no class." Dabbing her eyes with the tissue, she hurried to the front office as the door chime pealed its music three times in a row, announcing the first patients.

I grabbed my white lab coat from a wall peg as Donna hastily finished preparations for the scheduled visits. She smiled, holding a stack of charts, ready to call out those to place in exam rooms.

I draped my stethoscope about my neck. "One more thing before we start. Lydia Isaacs will be in today. I'll tell you both all about the dramatic house call on Monday if you share your holiday stories with me. I assume you girls had a picnic in the park with the famous Blackwell cousins."

Donna's face flushed. "You drive a hard bargain, but yes. We'll have a tell-all in exchange for another hilarious episode in the life of Lydia Isaacs."

CHAPTER 17—A FESTIVE OCCASION

*T*he following day in the office began with a promise of better things to come. Sunny skies and a temperature of seventy degrees with a gentle breeze from the west lifted my spirits. The changing season had already added a hint of fall coloring to the surrounding farms and woodlots. Jack O'Conner awaited me in exam room 1, the first patient of the day, and he was making amazing progress.

Donna handed me his chart with a smile and a flourish. "I can't wait to see what you think. Jack's vital signs are normal, and his color is excellent. Janie came with him today and made such a fuss over him he threatened to send her back to the waiting room. He's already over being waited on by family and friends and desperately wants to do everything for himself again."

Pulling out one report from his chart, I nodded. "Look at Dr. Stanberry's last office dictation. You're familiar with the cancer marker, CEA, aren't you?"

"I think so. Doesn't that stand for carcinoembryonic antigen?"

"That's right. When we get lucky, a positive test corelates to a gastrointestinal tumor like stomach carcinoma. It's still fairly new and doesn't always correlate with a specific carcinoma, but in his case, the results are very promising."

Donna quickly scanned the report before handing it back. "Wow. The CEA appeared extremely elevated before surgery. Now it's barely detectable. Is that accurate?"

"I think so. Dr. Stanberry had the same question and repeated the test with essentially the same result the second time." Flipping through the dictation, I showed Donna his response. "That has to be encouraging news."

"That's wonderful. Of course, you realize Christine won't give you any peace today until she's wrung out the last bit of information?"

"We'll face that when the time comes. You can run interference with her for now." Reaching for the exam room doorknob, I glanced back. "Don't let me down. Keep her busy this morning."

Donna threw her hands up, feigning distaste for the assignment. "Why me? What did I do wrong today?"

~

JACK AND JANIE sat at the far end of the room, relaxed and smiling. "Good morning. You two look chipper today."

Jack got up to extend a handshake, motioning toward the examination table. "Want me up there?"

"Sure. Slip your shirt off first, and we'll proceed."

Janie jumped up to help him remove his shirt, but he impatiently nodded toward her chair. "Please. Let me do this myself. I appreciate your help very much, but I need to care for myself as much as possible."

Embarrassed, Janie's cheeks reddened. "I'm only trying to help the man I love. I want to keep you around for a long time." She sat back down, not pushing the issue.

"Doc, my family is killing me with kindness. I can't even bend over to tie my shoes without one of them jumping up to do it for me. Janie still wants to serve me breakfast in bed. Lynn makes sure I have my slippers and morning newspaper, those items also brought first thing to the bedside. And William, now that's another story. I'm worried about him. It's September, and he's mowing the lawn three times a week so it'll 'look nice' for me. I keep asking him if he's wrecked my car or done something else equally horrible. He says no, but I have to wonder."

"He's getting better, Doc," Janie said. "He is grousing about everything, a sure sign of him getting back to normal. My husband's an action guy. Never sits still for long. Has to keep occupied. He's a natural as a mailman, joyfully walking his route for years, puttering in the garage after work, endless projects on his to-do list. The truth is, the rest of the family is hard pressed to keep up with him."

Seated on the examination table, Jack winked at Janie. "I relish giving them all a hard time. Keeps them off balance to my advantage. But I wouldn't trade a one of them for all the money in the world."

"Here's the report from Dr. Stanberry," I said. "Looks like he saw you a week ago. Is this a typo? He stated that you have no symptoms. Is that right?"

"Sure is. I feel back to normal, or I would if allowed to care for myself." He rolled his eyes at Janie.

"You have no post-op pain, no nausea, no constipation, no fever, nothing?"

"That about sums it up. Took my last pain pill two weeks ago. Like I told you before surgery, it's not my time to die. I think I'll know when that time comes." Jack paused, looking thoughtful for a few moments. "I'm not living in fantasy land, Doc. My diagnosis and treatment have given me a lot of time to think about life. The chemotherapy to date is more than tolerable. Doc Stanberry tells me I'm fortunate in that regard. I doubt that I'll reach a normal lifespan, but I've got some good years left to check off the important items on my to-do list that Janie mentioned. I'll be fine until I complete my goals."

"You're a man of great faith, my friend. The power of a positive attitude accompanied by prayer and thanksgiving is a powerful asset for recovering from a life-threatening illness."

Jack's physical examination was noteworthy for absence of abnormal findings. With a pleased, relaxed countenance, he dressed to leave. "It's a good sign that your examination is congruent with Dr. Stanberry's. Neither one of you found any sign of cancer, and my lab work is all normal. I'm doubly blessed for your help. Janie and I also want to especially thank you and the girls for insisting that Lynn get her application in for a scholarship to finish her college work." He finished buttoning his shirt. "That is a life-saver. Being sick has drained a considerable amount from my retirement since I had to cash in a fair amount early because of financial hardship. Thanks to everyone involved in the award process, Lynn won't have to give up her dreams."

Ready to leave, he held the door for Janie and chuckled. "I've a hunch another answer to my prayers is working out. Lynn can't talk five minutes without mentioning Paul Hawley. It's Paul said this, Paul plans to do that, Paul, Paul, Paul. They talked on the telephone three times last night. He's meeting her at House's Pharmacy at the soda fountain this afternoon 'to compare notes.' At least, that's what Lynn said was their motivation to meet. He's a year ahead of her and has some 'valuable pointers' to share for her last year of pre-med. I'm eager to meet him." Jack escorted Janie down the hallway, shaking his head and softly laughing.

∼

TIME PASSED UNEVENTFULLY as we finished the morning schedule for the day. Carrying a stack of charts, I retreated to the lounge table where I placed them to complete last details while eating my lunch.

Several moments passed and then I felt eyes boring into me. Startled, I looked up to find Christine on the other side of the table, arms folded, an impatient look on her face.

"Dr. Matlock, you know the drill. This girl cannot enjoy lunch without exhaustive knowledge regarding a special patient." She noisily cleared her throat. "You want me to be able to concentrate this afternoon, don't you?"

Trying to look nonchalant, I shrugged and remained silent.

Exasperated now, she leaned over, placing her palms on the tabletop, trying to assume a serious demeanor. "Well, don't you?"

Noticing Donna across the room with a wicked grin on her face, I shook my head. "You were supposed to help me keep her occupied. You're letting me down."

"Face it. She's hopeless and clueless."

Christine straightened up, hands on her hips. "Oh, you two. I have my reasons. It just so happens that I have to know how Jack's getting along. As a member of the ladies' planning committee at Reverend White's church, it's my responsibility to see if everything's a go for this Saturday evening."

Startled, I sat up and blinked. "You can't share patient information with the public."

Assuming a sweet tone of voice, Christine gave a slight nod as she continued, "My dearest friends, you both know I would never be guilty of such an indiscretion." She curtsied, then leaned down in my face. "Is Jack well enough to attend a party?"

Huffing, I scooted my chair away from the table and leaned back. "I give up. What do you need to know?"

Christine beamed as she yanked out a chair and sat down across from me. "Oh, goodie. I want—I mean, I need to know everything you can tell me. After all, Jack talks to me on the phone before he says a word to you or Donna. I need to know what to watch for regarding his appointments. And what's this CEA business?"

Christine sat in rapt attention as I explained and filled in the details.

Donna joined us as I finished the discussion, taking a seat at the end of the table. "A party sounds like fun. What occasion is the church celebrating for Jack?"

"My dear nurse, we're not only considering a celebration for Jack's recovery. We have a surprise party in mind to honor Lynn's achievement. I've already checked with Paul Hawley. He promised to make sure and deliver her to the shindig. What he can't know is that we plan to honor him as well. This is such fun."

"Christine, please don't tell me how you got the information to contact Paul. I don't think I want to know. That way I can plead innocent to all future charges."

"Relax, Doctor. I've already brought your exemplary wife into the conspiracy. We'll have a fine time. She's helping with the planning. And the icing on the cake: Marty Blackwell is off work Saturday and is bringing me."

Donna crossed her arms and leaned back. "A fine friend you are. That's not fair."

Christine's face lit up with a radiant smile. "I shouldn't tell you, but Jeff called to ask if I would mind if he invited you to go along on a double date with us to the party. He already cleared it with Marty, so I told him it was fine with me. That's what you would have wanted me to do, wasn't it?"

Donna looked relieved. "Yes. You really are a pal."

Christine stood up. "We'd better hurry to get lunch. Ethel House showed me the menu when I stopped by for donuts and coffee this morning. Her famous beef steak sandwich with all the trimmings and a slice of warm apple pie, a gourmet's delight."

The ladies locked the doors and hurried out chattering as I sat quietly, enjoying the sudden stillness and sense of calm pervading the office. I retrieved my hamburger from the refrigerator and popped it in the microwave. While it heated, I got ice from the dispenser and poured a Diet Coke. Although intending to enjoy the silence, I knew it wouldn't last long. Christine's departing words had put me on notice of the need to complete plans for the celebration the coming weekend. There would be no peaceful resolution until she had every detail nailed down to her satisfaction.

CHAPTER 18—THE CELEBRATION

*C*hristine and Donna continued zealously keeping the extravaganza a secret from those we wished to honor, and Saturday afternoon finally arrived. I had never seen Christine so close-mouthed around Lynn O'Conner in the past. It had to be a severe trial for her not to share her news. The ladies had spent hours calling and confirming invitations since Lynn and Paul both had to leave for their fall school semesters to begin on Monday, September 12. That gave no time for letters to be sent out.

Although formal dress was not required, I added a light-blue tie and a dark-blue sports jacket to my black slacks since I would say a few words about the scholarship selection. Rob Hendrick even planned to attend, representing the hospital as chairman of the committee.

The doorbell announced our babysitter for the evening, Marjorie House, Barry's and Ethel's youngest daughter. Janet finished combing her hair and stood to model for me. "How do I look?"

She took my breath away with her hair done up, a new blue dress, and black high heels. "Absolutely stunning." I congratulated myself on marrying such a beautiful and lovely lady as I gave her a quick kiss and grabbed the car keys off the nightstand. While Janet gave Marjorie last-minute instructions regarding snacks, playtime, and most importantly, bedtime, I hurried out to start the car.

The town hall center, a spacious meeting room, had been rented by the church because of the crowd expected to attend the event. I glanced at my watch. It was 4:30 already. Paul had promised to have Lynn there by 5:00 p.m. Marty Blackwell and Christine had one of Glen Oak's black-and-white police sedans washed and polished to escort the rest of the family to the event. Christine and Donna had finally advised the other family members about the gala party after office hours this morning. They still didn't know Jack was also being honored.

I looked over at Janet. "If those girls pull this off without spoiling the surprise, I'll be amazed. It'll probably be a first for Christine."

"You should have more confidence in them, dear," Janet said.

"I guess so. Anyway, we'll soon know."

~

ON ENTERING the town center building, I had to smile. Donna had Jeff Blackwell helping her set up a serving station at the far end of the room with an enormous punch bowl, cups, saucers, napkins, and silverware. An immense white frosted cake decorated with pink and blue flower designs adorned the center of the table. Packages of nuts and mints, soon to be placed in small cut glass bowls, awaited on a counter behind the table. Jeff appeared pleased to be helping Donna.

I nudged Janet. "Looks like Donna is doing all right. Jeff Blackwell acts like he's smitten with her."

Janet nodded. "He's lucky to be dating her. She looks so lovely in her pink dress and white heels. They look right together as a couple. I've got my fingers crossed for Donna."

The center filled up as guests arrived. Art McKay approached me, smiling and holding out his hand. "Good to see you, Doc and Mrs. Matlock. You think it will surprise Jack and Lynn?"

"We'll soon find out. They're due anytime now."

Ollie Stone brushed past us on the way to the refreshments while his partner, Willie Robertson, stopped to speak with Art and me. Willie exhaled and shook his head. "I told him to act like he has some manners tonight, even if it's an effort."

Art grinned. "He's a good boy under that rough exterior. We'll keep working with him. I'll try to stop him from eating all the nuts and mints before anyone else is served." With that, Art took off, hurrying to intercept his wayward EMT.

Willie crossed his arms, a sour look on his face. "Doc, you ever hear the saying 'you can't make a silk purse out of a sow's ear'?"

"I believe I've heard it."

"Well, Art's chasing the whole pig right now. Hopeless!"

Willie sauntered on to save a seat for the three of them. The room set-up featured four rows of tables, set parallel with the long side of the building, stretching nearly sixty feet per row. The serving tables where Jeff and Donna continued to set up at the far end were perpendicular to the long rows, while two tables for the guests of honor were at the opposite end beside the entrance, also facing perpendicular to the long rows.

I turned toward the entrance to watch people filing into the building when someone tapped me on the shoulder. It was the Donaldsons.

"Hello, Harvey. Good to see you, Emma," I said. "I'm glad both of you could make it tonight. It looks like we'll have a full house by the time we start."

Emma smiled as she clung to Harvey's arm. "Didn't want to miss meeting our new town doctor. I'm so pleased to meet you. We really need a doctor here. It's such a long way to the big city."

Harvey winked at me as he directed Emma to a seat. "Mom, Doc Matlock is already our doctor. We're here to celebrate Lynn's scholarship award."

She stopped walking and looked up at her son. "Lynn? Who's Lynn?"

With a patient look, Harvey took time to explain. "You know our neighbor, Lynn O'Conner. Her dad has been our mail carrier for years. Lynn will be a doctor someday soon."

"Do you have to stop by the post office now?"

He pulled out a chair and assisted her into it. "No, Mom. We're going to rest here a few minutes and have some refreshments. Please don't move while I go put our congratulation card in the basket with the others on the head table."

"Oh, dear. You do have a letter to mail. Don't worry, son. I'll wait here for you."

Harvey looked my way and shrugged helplessly as he made his way to add his greeting and small gift to the basket. Most of the townspeople had brought cards for Lynn and her father, with most even remembering to bring a card for Paul Hawley. This town had a heart for people.

Waiting for the guests of honor near the entrance, I looked about the room, trying to get an accurate count. I greeted Clayton and Bonita Harrison, closely followed by their daughter, Katy, and her husband, Michael Richardson. Next, my favorite fisherman, Johnny Morton, arrived with his date, Sherry House. She appeared to have landed him at last. Barry and Ethel House entered after them.

I grinned at Barry. "Who's minding the store tonight?"

"Don't worry about that, Doc. I got you covered. Closed up early for this, but you need anything for one of your patients, you only have to give me a nod."

Soon after, Lydia and Matilda Isaacs made their way into the room. Lydia surveyed the crowd expectantly, then shook my hand. "Sure is exciting. I hope I don't faint. I'm a little lightheaded already."

I pulled out a nearby chair for her. "We wouldn't want that to happen. You'd miss the celebration and the food."

Lydia, never one to suffer embarrassment about her expanding girth, considered that. "I would really hate to miss getting some cake and ice cream. And Jack O'Conner has been my mailman as long as I can remember. Do you think he'll be all right?"

"Lydia, you must talk to Jack to get his input. I can't give out that information without his consent."

"That's right. What's the matter with me? I know that, but you can tell anyone you want about my fainting spells. I have no secrets to hide. Goodness, but everyone here has witnessed one of my spells at one time or another."

Stifling a laugh, I offered my hand to help her up. Matilda thanked me and ushered her mother to a spot farther down the row.

Nearly five o'clock and they were all here: Ann Kilgore and her husband, Sally and Russell Christopher, Jack's fishing buddies, our entertaining town gossip Laura Dawson, and too many more friends and neighbors to mention.

Just before 5:00, Rob Hendrick hurried in the door and greeted me. "Am I late?"

"No, the guests of honor are pulling into the reserved parking spot now. My office assistant, Christine, and her boyfriend, Marty Blackwell, picked up Jack, Janie, and their son William. Marty is driving one of the squad cars and Tom Collins, our town marshal, is leading the parade. Paul Hawley is driving the third car. He surprised Lynn by bringing her here for their date. I'm told she had no clue about tonight."

Rob beamed. "Paul will get a surprise when he learns the celebration is in his honor too."

"Yes, he'll be shocked. I believe my office staff kept this event a surprise. That may be their most unbelievable accomplishment."

～

THE EVENT SUCCEEDED beyond our expectations. The surprise was complete. The meal with ham and beef cold-cut sandwiches, potato salad, chips, and a relish tray was delicious. Punch and generous slabs of cake served with vanilla ice cream were special favorites with everyone. Watching the interactions around the room during the time of fellowship, listening to conversations between lifelong friends, seeing smiles on many faces, I knew why I had become a country doctor. The rewards from hard work in a community of people with shared values far exceeded my expectations. Rural Americans are still some of my favorite people on earth.

The extemporaneous speeches by Paul and Lynn were brief, heartfelt, and filled with praise for the people of Glen Oaks. When Jack finished his turn speaking, there were few dry eyes in the room. It was a night to be remembered by all.

At 8:00, Lynn and Paul left hand in hand to warm applause and a few shrill wolf whistles. Christine and Marty drove Jack and the rest of his family home shortly afterward. Jeff and Donna began cleaning up while the church youth group pitched in, some folding and stacking chairs and tables out of the way while others swept the floors.

In about fifteen minutes, Christine and Marty returned to help with the clean-up. Janet and I offered to help finish the chores, but Marty said, "Go on home, Doc. We can finish up here." He then turned and tossed his car keys to Jeff, saying, "How would you like to take a cruise in the squad car? Tom said you could drive it. I think he wants to recruit you for a second deputy."

"With the girls?" Jeff asked.

"Naturally, cousin. Naturally. I'm thinking of a late-night stroll through the park."

Jeff looked at Donna. "In that case, you're on. Right, ladies?"

Christine and Donna answered, "Right."

And so ended a perfect evening.

CHAPTER 19—TIMELY REFLECTIONS

October arrived with a new coolness in the air as trees and shrubs turned into a gorgeous panorama of color with shades of orange, red, yellow, and brown along with a fading tint of green, all liberally dispensed from God's palette of nature. Yards and pastures near town took on a yellow-brown hue following an early killing frost.

On a one-hundred-acre tract a few miles from my office, golden-brown corn stalks loaded with ripened ears bowed gently in the wind as a giant green John Deere combine harvester took long swathes, spewing out stripped corncobs and cornstalks in the rear. Dust rose slowly in the air, marking the path of the harvester when it worked the far side of the field.

I sat mesmerized, watching from the window of my car parked off the side of the road as the unchallenged green titan came back into view, powerful engine throbbing, intermittently filling grain wagons hauled by separate tractors, golden-yellow grain flowing like a fountain from the long funnel of the unloader on the harvester. As soon as one wagon filled up, it departed with a load of grain for transport by semi to storage bins nearby, while another tractor-grain wagon combination quickly took its place.

Saturday afternoon already, and I could watch this all day but for the long to-do list on the seat beside me. Taking a deep breath, I restarted my car and headed back to town. Fast-paced and hectic morning clinic now behind me and my house call completed, my stomach reminded me of the need for nourishment. Glancing at my watch, I noted the time: 1:22 p.m. No food since a hurried bite at 5:00 a.m. when I got up to deliver a baby.

With my wife and children visiting relatives in southern Indiana for the weekend, I needed to get to Barry House's store before 1:30. Ethel quit serving lunch then. Fortunately, Glen Oaks was only five miles away.

∾

BREATHLESS AFTER AN UNDIGNIFIED run from my car parked a block down the street and just beating the deadline, I hurried to take a seat in a booth near the lunch bar, nodding at Ethel as I picked up the menu. She and two of her daughters, Sherry and Marjorie, waited on two customers before me. At last, Ethel came around the counter to greet me. "What'll it be, Doc? We got you covered. We planned to hold lunch open for you anyway, so relax. Christine and Donna ate here and left a few minutes ago. They made sure I knew you'd be in since your family is out of town. We have to take care of our town doctor."

I should have known. "Thanks, Ethel. I appreciate your kindness."

"Those girls who work for you are the ones to thank. They're very thoughtful young ladies. So, do you want the usual?"

"Sure. Make it a hamburger with dill pickles and a Diet Coke. This time add a cup of coffee. I've been up since five and I'm not finished with my day yet. I have a stack of supplemental insurance forms for patients that need my personal attention this afternoon. After that, back to the hospital to dictate charts and check on a new admission."

"Coming right up. The girls will bring your coffee over right away while I get your sandwich with all the trimmings on the side ready. Just made a fresh pot of coffee. Sodas, malts, soft drinks, coffee, and potato chips are available all day anyway." She handed me a copy of the Glen Oaks newspaper. "Here, read this while you wait. You'll get a kick out of it. Laura Dawson's gossip column is hysterical today. I still don't know whatever possessed them to allow her to write that column of weekly baloney. She writes well, but not a word is believable. I'm still sore at her for writing that I hit Barry over the head with one of our frying pans. She was here in the store when a bucket of paint fell off a top shelf and struck the top of his head. From there, the story grew until she had me attacking him with bodily harm in mind." Ethel motioned to Sherry and then pointed to the coffee pot.

Sherry hurried over with a cup. "Made the way you like it, Doc. Strong, hot, and black. How are you today?"

"I'm fine, only a little tired. Nothing a few hours of sleep won't remedy. By the way, how are you and Johnny Morton getting along these days?"

"You mind if I sit down for a minute?" Without waiting for my answer, she scooted into the seat across from me. "I'd like some advice about Johnny."

"What kind of advice?"

"Well, I'm playing second fiddle to his obsession with fishing too often." She leaned forward and rested her elbows on the table, lowering her voice in a conspiratorial manner.

"How can I help you with that? I don't believe I qualify to give advice about romance."

"Sure you do. You know Johnny, and you know me. You like to fish. You know how men think."

I shrugged my shoulders, not knowing where this conversation led.

"I've tried flirting and flattery, but nothing works when he gets the urge to go fishing. My plan is to feign an interest in learning to fish. Actually, I think I'll hate it. I don't like killing animals, but I'm exceptionally good at pretending. Do you think he'll fall into my little trap?"

Chuckling now, I struggled to stifle a laugh. "Well, you won't have to pretend."

Sherry raised her eyebrows and looked surprised. "Whatever do you mean by that?"

"You've got to admit, Johnny's a pretty big catch. Seems to me you'll be fishing for something besides an animal that lives in the water."

"Oh, Doc. You're impossible. I'm serious about wanting help." Sherry leaned back in the seat and folded her arms across her chest.

"And I gave you a serious answer. I'm sure if you roll your eyes exactly right, cast your line into a tree two or three times, and give him a helpless look, he'll be glad to put his arm around you and steady your pole while teaching you to cast for fish. You might even repeat the bad cast until he finally gets the hint."

Sherry put her hand over her mouth, trying not to laugh. Then she smiled. "That's a great idea. I knew you'd help me. I will land that big hunk if it's the last thing I do."

Ethel brought my lunch with added chips plus tomato and lettuce on the side. "What are you doing bothering Doc? Get back behind the counter so he can eat in peace. It's your turn to clean up the grill and fryer today."

"I'm on it, Mom. But I wasn't bothering him. He's been giving me the most wonderful advice about how to win Johnny Morton's love and affection." Sherry sped off to finish working.

Ethel shook her head in disbelief. "Did you actually give her advice about her love life with Johnny?"

"Must have. She said that's what happened, although I was mostly joking with her about applying her charms on him. I told her in advance that I'm not qualified to give advice regarding her love life."

Now it was Ethel's turn to take a seat across from me. "I trust you, but do you mind telling me about the advice that you 'didn't give' Sherry? I may have to deal with her if she's about to do something stupid. She has an overactive imagination as it is."

So I had to repeat the entire story to Ethel's satisfaction before taking a bite from my hamburger, which had now grown cold.

Afterward, Ethel got up and picked up my plate. "I'm sorry. I'll warm this up for you. And I can't believe Sherry thought you were serious. Wait until I get through with her for disturbing your meal."

"Sherry's a delightful girl, full of fun and with big dreams. Don't be too hard on her for my sake. She probably knew I was joking, as much as she laughed afterward. She won't do anything to disgrace you. When he finally grows up, Johnny Morton will make a great husband and father. Remember, Sherry's fishing, using her feminine wiles as bait, but still, she's fishing, like Johnny. Only he's the desired catch."

Ethel shook her head and chuckled. "You're right about her. She's a good girl. She and Johnny make a handsome couple. I wouldn't be all that upset if she succeeds in her quest. Enough of this. I'll be right back with your warmed food."

After finishing lunch, I folded the newspaper and placed it on the table for the next customer, left a tip, and paid Ethel at the counter. "A fine lunch, as usual. Your sandwiches are better than any in Glen Falls."

Ethel smiled in appreciation. "Glad you enjoyed it. Try to have a good rest of the day."

～

As I TURNED TO LEAVE, a tap on my shoulder got my attention. "Hey, Doc, got a minute?"

I turned. "Hello, Jack. It's fantastic to see you up and around. Looks like you got your medication refilled today."

He nodded. "These nausea pills are a great relief after chemotherapy treatments. But I'm doing okay otherwise. Doc Stanberry says that he's found no sign of recurrent cancer."

"That's wonderful. What can I do for you?"

"I'm getting my exercise today. Do you feel like a short walk?"

Considering my afternoon schedule, I hesitated until noticing the hopeful expression on Jack's face. "Sure thing. Let's do it."

Crossing the street, we strolled up Main Street past the bank and headed for the small park two blocks away. Jack tolerated the walk with no lagging but pointed to one of the park benches when we arrived. "Mind if we sit and talk a minute?"

The sun illuminated the beautiful changing leaves of the oaks and maples in the park, and the temperature had moderated, climbing to the mid-seventies. "It's been a hectic day. I could use a few minutes of rest too."

For a couple of minutes, Jack sat in silence as we enjoyed the beauty of nature. At last, he looked at me. "You and your office have been very kind to me and my family."

"We just did our job in taking care of you."

"No, now wait. I believe in handing out bouquets while I'm still alive." He shrugged. "You and your staff deserve our unending gratitude."

I faced forward, pretending not to notice the tear that he quickly wiped from his cheek. He choked up but only briefly. "And this wonderful town of Glen Oaks. The surprise party took my breath away. We love this town and its people."

Not sure what to say, choked up myself, I nodded.

Jack smiled as I turned my head, making eye contact again. "God is answering my prayers. I'm not naïve enough to believe the cancer won't come back, but I've asked for five more years to live. I fully expect to make that goal."

"I'll pray that you have five plus years, my friend."

"Five will be enough, Doc. I want to see Lynn graduate from medical school and that'll take five more years of study and hard work, but I know she'll make it through. After that, I want to walk her down the aisle and give her away, hopefully to Paul. What a beautiful bride and handsome groom they'll be on their wedding day."

"How is that romance coming?"

"Just fine. Paul doesn't let any grass grow under his feet. There's a young man of action. I think he wanted to be sure she didn't develop an interest in someone else in her last year of college. He asked her to be his steady girlfriend." He paused, laughing under his breath. "I proposed to

Janie on our second date. She nearly bowled me over. She said yes and here we are, still happily married."

"Well, how did Lynn answer him?"

"She accepted, of course. After avoiding long-term relationships while pursuing her dreams, that young man just swept her away. I've never seen Lynn happier. The good Lord is helping her find her way. I'm convinced of that."

"I'm sure you're right."

"Another thing. I don't regret developing cancer."

A shocking statement that took me by surprise. "Seriously?"

"Seriously. If I hadn't developed cancer, I would have had the financial means of supporting her through medical school. She wouldn't have needed a scholarship, and she might never have met Paul."

"That's a wonderful perspective. I'm glad you've found peace about your health and the future for your daughter."

"There's also William to consider. You wouldn't recognize him as the same young man prior to my diagnosis. He's taken an interest in church and can't do enough for the family these days. He's accepted Jesus in his life, and that alone would make my illness worth it all."

Unable to speak, I patted him on the knee.

"One last thing. The Lord has given me time to prepare financially for Janie when I'm gone. I met with my financial planner and mapped out the future. We set everything to provide for her needs when the time comes." Jack looked up at the lazy cumulus clouds floating overhead, a smile on his face. "Know something, Doc? God gives hope and light in the darkest night of despair we poor humans face. I wouldn't trade the peace I have for the promise of living to be one hundred years old."

We got up and walked back to Main Street. On arriving at my car, I shook hands with him. "You've given me a great slogan to remember, hope and light in the darkest night. Your life is a great blessing to many. Don't ever change. This town loves you and your family a lot. I believe God will answer your prayers."

Jack nodded. "I know, Doc. I know."

CHAPTER 20—SEVEN YEARS LATER

*J*une 1984 arrived in Glen Oaks with blue skies, fluffy white clouds floating overhead, and hot weather. On a beautiful Saturday morning, I drove into town from the north on Main Street and noticed Jack rocking in his front porch swing waving at me. With time to spare before office hours, I swung the car to the curb and parked.

Joining Jack on the porch, I smiled at realizing he had his first grandson, little Paul Junior, in his arms. The front screen door opened, and Lynn and Paul came out to greet me. "Good morning, Jack, and the Doctors Hawley and family," I said. "It's great to see you."

Jack's face reflected peace and joy. "Thanks for stopping, Doc. It's time you met my grandson, Paul Hawley Junior. He's already a handsome charmer, isn't he?"

"May I?" I reached for the baby.

"You'd better. He's my pride and joy." Jack handed him over while Lynn and Paul stood beside me admiring little Paul.

"How's everything coming with the office in Glen Falls?"

Paul grinned. "Just great. The office furniture will arrive next week. I plan to open my practice the first week of July. I really appreciate the advice you've given me on getting set up." Paul had completed his residency in family practice in May and was ready to start. Lynn had one year to go in her family practice residency at Methodist Hospital in Indianapolis. The couple planned to live in an apartment in suburban Indianapolis until she finished training and joined Paul in practice in another year.

We visited a few minutes until Paul Junior became fussy and his parents took him back inside for a diaper change and a visit with Grandma. I sat down on the stone porch railing, exchanging idle talk with Jack until it was time to leave for the office. Glancing at my watch, I stood up to leave.

"It was good of you to stop by, Doc. Before you go, did you get the latest reports on me from Dr. Stanberry?"

I nodded. "They came in the mail earlier this week."

"Then you know. My cancer's back. Been losing a little weight, but my appetite's still good. There isn't much pain so far. I'm not sure whether or not to accept another round of chemotherapy. What would you do?"

"It's difficult to answer that. What did Dr. Stanberry say about the chances of a remission again?"

"That's just it. There's less than a fifty-fifty chance of success."

Nodding, I took his hand in a firm grip. "I know. Just wanted to be sure you understood the odds. The truth is that no one can answer that for you. He indicated that more chemotherapy could make you seriously ill. It might even shorten your life more than withholding treatment. Still, there's a chance of success if you decide to proceed."

Jack slowly stood up, shakily taking my hand again for support. He appeared frail and weak compared to the robust man I had known for so long. "Remember our conversation in the park several years ago?"

"How could I ever forget? You taught me about hope in the darkness. Your courage in this fight against cancer is truly inspiring."

"Well, Doctor, I'm tired of fighting. I hate to leave my family behind, but I have a mom, dad, and other loved ones waiting for me on the other side. I'm ready to put on immortality, as the Good Book says. Besides, all my family are now ready to meet me in God's tomorrow. That's all that really counts in this life."

"You're so right about that, Jack." I gripped his hand one last time before departing for the office. "Whatever you decide, the office staff and I will be there for you. This is not a battle you'll face alone."

Jack smiled and put up his right hand in an expressive wave as I descended the porch steps. "Just remember. God gives hope and light in the darkest night of the soul. Life, real life, is just a little way ahead for me, and for all believers."

NOTES

Chapter 3–Never a Boring Moment

1. In those days, we didn't have access to ultrasound for pregnancy diagnosis, and the fetoscope was a long trumpet-like device that the doctor attached to his head with a metal frame to hold it in place while listening through the earpieces. In that way, sound transmitted to the examiner by both the ears and bone conduction through the headpiece. Those stethoscopes, now assigned to the dustbin of medical history in the United States, now exist only in museums and collections of elderly physicians who practiced OB.

Chapter 13—Chaos in the Office

1. Michael and Katy's story is told in *Until Shadows Flee Away: A Country Doctor's Story of Christmas Seasons Past.*

AUTHOR'S NOTE

I hope you enjoyed this book. It's entirely a work of fiction but is based on my experiences of practicing both family and emergency medicine for forty-seven years. For those who doubt that a cancer patient with a dire prognosis can survive so long, one of my father's sisters, my Aunt Ruby, lived for more than twenty years after experiencing invasive metastatic carcinoma. And she turned down anything but local excision.

During my career, I had the privilege of caring for several cancer patients on hospice who had to be taken off the service because they refused to die. Hospice patients are theoretically expected to have a survival time of six months or less. One of the interesting findings in working with various hospice groups is that they often prolong the life of the patient, so much so that the patient may require termination from the program. The goal of hospice is to relieve end-of-life pain and suffering, along with providing spiritual nurturing and emotional support. When these goals are met, some patients become so relaxed mentally and emotionally that they far exceed their expected survival date. Some live productive lives for quite a while after hospice.

In treating hundreds of patients who developed cancer, I found a few common denominators for survival. In no particular order of importance, these include early diagnosis, a positive outlook, a will to fight for life, and a strong faith in God. On the other hand, patients who lacked most of these qualities rarely lasted long in their battle. I always hated to hear a patient give up, as life for them was usually brief.

In telling these stories, names, sexes, geographic locations, and many other factors have frequently been changed. Multiple character traits and flaws of several patients were often combined in one fictional person in the story. In other cases, a colorful character was represented by up to three or more fictional people. Some of my characters are so make-believe that they exist only in my imagination. I give this detailed explanation in response to a reviewer who questioned whether I had gotten valid permissions from my fictional characters. I want to assure the reader that no living or deceased person has been identified in the storyline.

During my career, I was privileged to treat thousands of delightful patients. We didn't refer to them as clients in my day. My characters are a composite of thousands of individuals, but not one identifiable person.

To answer another question, did these types of events really happen? Did I practice for a time in a modern-day Mayberry? The short answer is a resounding yes. Also, the stories about my wife and children are real, although not necessarily in the exact sequence of events in our lives. My wife contributed tremendously to my ability to practice medicine. Always patient with me and caring toward those who called me their doctor, she provided the emotional support to make my sometimes-overwhelming life as a doctor possible.

This story was inspired by the powerful response of many individuals who refused to give up in the face of overwhelming odds. It has been my privilege to know and to learn from such inspiring fighters. If the reader is experiencing an overwhelming battle with cancer, depression, financial stress, family crisis, or anything else imaginable, please take heart. I really do believe there is light and hope in the darkest night of despair when God is honored and placed first in life.

Thanks again for reading.

Carl K. Matlock, MD

ALSO BY CARL MATLOCK MD

Medical

1. The Annals of a Country Doctor

2. Reminiscence: Life of a Country Doctor

3. Until Shadows Flee Away, A Country Doctor's Story of Christmas Seasons Past

Biblical Fiction

1. Rebel Against the Eagle – available only as first edition paperback.

2. Rebels, Romans, and the Rabbi, A Story of Jewish Romance, Rebellion, and Reconciliation – available only as eBook. (**Revised edition of *Rebels against the Eagle*).**

3. Jerusalem Crucible – Available in paperback and eBook format.

Dear Reader,

I hope you enjoyed my latest book. If you would like to be advised of future releases, please visit my web page at https://www.carlmatlockmd.com, and hit the subscribe button to receive my newsletter. My e-mail is doctorcarl@carlmatlockmd.com . I am beginning work on my fifth book in the family practice medical series and will keep you informed of its availability.

My books are all listed on Amazon.com. I hope you enjoy reading them as much as I do in writing them. I can be reached on Facebook at Carl Matlock MD / Author. Comments are welcome and book reviews on Amazon are especially appreciated.

Made in the USA
Monee, IL
29 October 2021